Advances in Mental Health and Addiction

Series Editor

Masood Zangeneh, Richmond Hill, Canada

Over the past several decades we have witnessed dramatic shifts in prevailing approaches to mental health and addiction. Significant scientific achievements have led to novel treatment options that impacted the experiences of individuals with mental disorders. In recent years, new perspectives have begun to influence the way we address mental health and substance dependencies, resulting in a greater emphasis on mental health promotion and prevention strategies. Despite these progressions, mental health care systems too often remain stagnant, fragmented, and peripheral.

Augusto Pérez-Gómez • Juliana Mejía-Trujillo
Editors

Drug Abuse Prevention

A Global Approach

Springer

Editors
Augusto Pérez-Gómez
Corporación Nuevos Rumbos
Bogotá, Colombia

Juliana Mejía-Trujillo
Corporación Nuevos Rumbos
Bogotá, Colombia

ISSN 2570-3390 ISSN 2570-3404 (electronic)
Advances in Mental Health and Addiction
ISBN 978-3-031-99620-7 ISBN 978-3-031-99621-4 (eBook)
https://doi.org/10.1007/978-3-031-99621-4

This Springer imprint is published by the registered company Springer Nature Switzerland AG
The registered company address is: Gewerbestrasse 11, 6330 Cham, Switzerland

Introduction

In 2015, the editors of this book, together with Professor Elisardo Becoña, from the Santiago de Compostela University in Spain, invited 21 researchers from nine countries to participate in the publication of a book titled "On prevention and other stories: History and evolution of the prevention of alcohol and drug consumption in Latin America and Europe." The book was widely disseminated throughout the continent and became a reference source for those working in this field.

But time goes on. Almost 10 years have passed and situations have evolved, for better or worse, in many countries. So, we considered important to do a review of what was happening in different parts of the world, and that is why we sent invitations to researchers from more than 20 countries, with the purpose of being able to compare what was happening on all continents. However, we did not receive a response from any African or Asian country, so we had to change the original title, "Prevention in the world," to the current one: "Drug abuse prevention: a global approach."

In this book there are big changes compared to the 2015 one: there is a chapter on the United States, one on Turkey and one on Australia, which did not appear in the previous version; a global chapter on Europe; three chapters from Latin American countries (Argentina, Colombia, and Mexico); one on the implementation of a preventive program in Brazil and Argentina; and one on the importance of evaluating preventive programs.

Roberto Canay and María Verónica Brasesco examine in detail the evolution of public policies on drugs in Argentina and take a look at the different areas of prevention, among which the community, work, education, and actions with people deprived of their rights stand out freedom. The authors present a critique of policy instability and lack of investment, which is probably a common feature of many Latin American countries. They also show that there are very few evaluations of preventive programs.

John Toumbourou and his colleagues in Australia show how important public policy decisions have been made over the years to ensure better health in relation to tobacco, alcohol, and other substances, especially among young people. Likewise, they have developed strategies based on the identification of protective and risk factors, insisting on the management of environmental conditions, quality of food, and programs in schools and with families. Australia's developments have had a significant influence on countries in the region known as the Asia Pacific. There are longitudinal studies in the country that allow monitoring the effectiveness of interventions.

In Colombia, Augusto Pérez-Gómez and Juliana Mejía-Trujillo take a look at the evolution of public policies since 1920 and make a description of prevention actions in the country, few of which have high-quality evaluations. Likewise, they analyze publications on prevention from 2015, pointing out that most of them are related to prevalence of consumption of different substances. There is no global analysis that explains what is happening in the country, which is characterized, like Argentina, by the lack of state policies, which leads to each change of government abandoning what the previous one could have attempted.

Elisardo Becoña and Amador Calafat make a successful attempt to synthesize what is happening in the different countries of Europe, and show that, even though there are specific initiatives in each one, there is an important similarity with regard to public policies on drugs and alcohol consumption, and the way to address, prevent and treat the problem. Furthermore, harm reduction strategies have been developed, especially since the emergence of HIV/AIDS, since in Europe one of the main sources of infection of this virus was associated with injected heroin.

José Luis Benítez and Carmen Fernández focus on explaining the models for addressing the drug problem in Mexico; and then they show what type of preventive programs are used in different settings—community, school, family—several of which have already been formally evaluated. In this sense, Mexico is a good example to follow for the rest of the continent.

Murat Yildirim and colleagues from Türkiye show that recent years have seen important reforms in legal regulations and preventive interventions. Traditionally, the country had adopted a criminological and punitive approach, but currently it tends to be much more similar to European countries, as it has preventive and rehabilitative programs in which both public and private organizations intervene.

William Crano, Eusebio Alvaro, and Jason Siegel comprehensively explain the evolution of preventive campaigns in the United States, a country that was not only a pioneer in this field (the first attempts date back to the end of the nineteenth century), but also became a model for all other countries for their efforts to refine concepts, improve approaches, evaluate interventions and, finally, give way to what is known today as "prevention science."

Maria Elena Ituarriaga (Argentina), Thaís Pereira, and Telmo Ronzani (Brazil) show the results of a process of adaptation of one of the most well-known and used prevention programs, Life Skills, in Argentina and Brazil. Even though it is a qualitative evaluation and recognizes the absence of quantitative data on the changes produced by the program as a limitation, it provides interesting data on these processes and contributes to a better understanding of their potential in diverse scenarios.

Finally, Orlando Scoppetta, from Colombia, gives a vision on the evaluation of prevention programs in the twenty-first century, ensuring that a program without evaluation may be a program, but not prevention. He describes the types of evaluation according to their purpose, shows the different levels of evidence that a program can have, and the evaluation trends at the current time.

We hope readers around the world will find this book not only interesting and helpful but also inspiring in continuing prevention efforts in their own countries.

APG and JMT, editors

Contents

Strategies and Policies for the Prevention of Substance Consumption in Argentina

Roberto Canay and Maria Veronica Brasesco

Country Context

Argentina is a country in South America that adopts republican, democratic, representative, and federal forms of government. It is organized as a federal state, decentralized, and integrated since 1994 for 23 provinces and the Autonomous City of Buenos Aires (CABA), the federal capital of the country. According to the last census (2022), the country's total population is 46,044,703. Its area is 2,780,400 km^2, making Argentina the eighth country with the largest area globally (National Institute of Statistics and Census of Argentina, 2024). The official religion is Catholic, and the language is Spanish. The country's economy is based on agriculture, livestock, industry, and commerce.

Introduction

Latin America, as the regional context of Argentina, is one of the regions with the greatest inequalities in the world. Inequality is expressed in the lack of access to social and health goods and services, as well as in relation to gender, age, ethnicity, and many other conditions. In this framework, drug policy in Argentina presents

R. Canay (✉)
ITTC Argentina, Instituto Forum Vitae de la Obra Social Ferroviaria, Universidad del Museo Social Argentino, Ciudad Autónoma de Buenos Aires, Autónoma de Buenos Aires, Argentina

Consultants, Synergy Group, Buenos Aires, Argentina

M. V. Brasesco
ISSUP Argentina, Universidad del Museo Social Argentino, Ciudad Autónoma de Buenos Aires, Autónoma de Buenos Aires, Argentina

A. Pérez-Gómez, J. Mejía-Trujillo (eds.), *Drug Abuse Prevention*, Advances in Mental Health and Addiction, https://doi.org/10.1007/978-3-031-99621-4_1

multiple challenges, having as a general characteristic the wide gap that exists between the quantity and quality of the offer of services and programs on the one hand, and the magnitude of substance consumption on the other, where both sectoral and more transversal problems stand out (Canay and Brasesco, 2014).

Regarding sectoral problems, the following stand out: shortcomings in the education and health sectors, particularly in certain regions; poor contributory social security coverage; disorderly increase and ineffective management of targeted programs. Regarding the unresolved problems of transversality, it is worth mentioning at least the following: lack of comprehensiveness of the interventions, associated with lack of coordination at the inter-sectoral and interjurisdictional level; weakness of state oversight (at its different levels) in the presence of new actors from the market, civil society, and the international system; discontinuity of the national state to promote training and equitable resources in the national territory and insufficiency and inefficiency in the distribution and execution of spending destined for the prevention and treatment of substance consumption.

Such characterization emphasizes the negative features without implying ignoring the virtues and potential that the Argentine public welfare system still possesses and aims to inscribe the problems of drug policy in general, and those linked to the decentralization of services and programs in particular, in a broader context.

This section attempts to analyze and debate history to think about the future of Public Policies on Addictions (with a focus on prevention) in Argentina, encouraging the installation of a broad and open debate so that all sectors of society become aware of the various aspects of the problems associated with substance consumption and other addictive behaviors, contributing to the strengthening of municipal, provincial, national, and regional strategies (Ministry of Justice, 2016; Wrobel, 2006).

Drug policy in Argentina in the last 90 years has taken multiple and contradictory directions. In the 1920s, drug consumption prevailed in the upper classes and was considered a criminal act that should be prosecuted by the police. This repressive vision of intervention to address the phenomenon of drug consumption persisted until the 1960s, when Argentina (1963) ratified the Single Convention on Narcotic Drugs of 1961 (UNODC, 2013).

In 1968, Law 19.567 was passed, which exempted the possession of drugs for personal use from criminal sanctions, strengthening both the Ethical-Legal model and the Medical-Sanitary model (Nowlis 1982; Parga, 2016). From the police field, the first national anti-drug network was formed in collaboration with international organizations, and from the therapeutic field, the Toxicological Aid Fund—FAT (Camarotti and Güelman, 2018), the first institution specialized in treatment and rehabilitation, was created, dependent on the Chair of Toxicology of the Faculty of Medicine of the University of Buenos Aires. This last initiative was accompanied from a legislative point of view with a reform of the Civil Code that allowed the disqualification and mandatory hospitalization of "drug addicts."

The 1970s are an important turning point, where the idea begins to prevail that, in the problem of consumption, the weight does not fall only on the person or on the substances, but that there is a third fundamental element, which is the social context and cultural where it is consumed.

In 1971, the international control system was extended to substances in the pharmaceutical industry. The Drug Addiction Service is created at the Borda Hospital, and in 1972 the National Commission on Drug Addiction and Narcotics (CONATON) (General Archive of the Argentine Nation, 2024) is created, dependent on the Ministry of Social Welfare, whose function was to advise the government executive. The composition of the Commission is interesting, which indicates a change in the vision of consumption as a multidimensional phenomenon, being made up of representatives of the Ministry of Social Welfare, Justice, Education, Foreign Affairs and Worship, Labor, Defense, Federal Police, Secretariat of State Information (SIDE), and the University of Buenos Aires.

Within this context, where consumption is seen as a social mental health issue that impacts public safety and necessitates re-education, the National Center for Social Reeducation (CENARESO), also known as the National Reference Center in Mental Health, was established in 1973, today called the National Hospital for Mental Health and Addictions, dependent on the National Mental Health Directorate. This institution was emblematic of the changes in the addiction care model, and in the 1980s the pedagogical model began to be abandoned for a more clearly social clinical model.

In the 1990s, with the emergence of HIV associated with injectable drug use, this institution incorporated a clinical analysis unit and also incorporated work on social reintegration within the treatment space. In the last two years, since the enactment of the Mental Health Law (Honorable Congress of the Argentine Nation, 2010), a purely social reading of the problem prevails, emphasizing social vulnerability and the rights approach in care: primary health and community care.

It should be noted that since 1983 with the return to democracy, work began on prevention tasks understood as a health problem and when the Programming Secretariat for the Prevention of Drug Addiction and the Fight against Drug Trafficking—SEDRONAR, was created. Through Decree 271/89 (Gil, 2022), the notion of the necessary comprehensiveness of a drug policy with inter-sectoral coordination and coordination between the reduction of supply and the reduction of demand is already installed. At SEDRONAR, the Consumption Prevention Directorate[1] becomes one of the three-pillar directorates along with Assistance[2] and Drug Trafficking.[3]

In 1989, Law 23,737 punishes the possession of substances, but with options for preventive and curative penalties (Ministry of Health, sf). More specifically, if the

---

[1] In terms of Prevention, it designs, executes, and supervises national programs and plans, referring to the prevention and training of community agents, on the subject of drug and alcohol abuse and its consequences, throughout the country, with the consensus and cooperation of governmental and non-governmental organizations.

[2] In terms of Assistance, it seeks to facilitate the help and rehabilitation of people who abuse or depend on drugs, and who, lacking adequate resources, could not access the treatment or recovery they deserve.

[3] In the fight against drug trafficking, it coordinates at the national level information and strategies aimed at detecting and disrupting the trade and distribution of illegal drugs.

person presents incipient consumption, the preventive measure is applied, with the sense of raising awareness of the personal and community impact of consumption or the curative measure (when the person is addicted), understood as a coercive rehabilitation treatment by the substance consumption. Despite certain shortcomings of this regulation, it is important to recognize that the implementation of this law allowed access to treatment to numerous addicts from impoverished sectors who were unaware of the possibility and scope of said treatments.

Based on the need to design and apply evidence-based drug policies, in 1999 SEDRONAR carried out the first national survey on drug consumption, where it is estimated that around 600,000 people use drugs throughout the country and 200,000 frequently (Gil, 2022). This first survey was the foundation of what would become the Argentine Drug Observatory in 2002, in charge of diagnosing and carrying out epidemiological surveillance of substance consumption in dissimilar settings such as school, health, work, etc. (CICAD, 2010).

In those first years, investment in prevention was always very little and actions were limited to campaigns based on occurrences, without any type of evaluation or data to support channels, content, or target population. Some of these campaigns were known for their slogans "Damn cocaine," or for their novel ideas such as "Fleco y Male" (the name of two cartoons that talked about ecstasy).

During the following years, SEDRONAR gives federal impetus to community participation based on evidence in addiction prevention, with the Local Studies Centers Program—CEL (in agreement with the National Council for Scientific and Technical Research—CONICET). At the end of the 1990s, 50 CELs located throughout the national territory were created and trained in research and for the first time there was information (scientific evidence) in the health, educational, and community spheres on drug consumption to design preventive programs according to the needs of each local area.

Starting in 2001, some provincial drug observatories began to be created with their own budget. The provinces of La Pampa, Córdoba, and the Autonomous City of Buenos Aires stand out, where the culture of research and the programming of policies and actions based on their own information are consolidated. In 2010, the Drug Observatory of the Autonomous City of Buenos Aires held the First Argentine Congress of Public Policies on Addictions, a space that focuses on public policies and community prevention strategies based on evidence.

Depending on the commitments assumed internationally by Argentina (UN-OAS), and the national regulations regarding the drug problem, there is a series of guiding principles that guide the strategies, objectives, and actions of public policies on drugs, having ratified the three UN conventions (1961, 1971, and 1988). It should be noted that what was postulated in these conventions was reaffirmed by the Inter-American Commission against Drug Abuse in May 2010 and by the Statute of the South American Council on the World Drug Problem of the Union of South American Nations (UNASUR) (National Executive Branch, 1996).

SEDRONAR, currently called the Secretariat of Comprehensive Drug Policies of the Argentine Nation, in its capacity as the agency for the implementation of national efforts to confront the different aspects that constitute the Argentine drug problem, has the obligation to prepare and approve a "Federal Comprehensive Drug Prevention Plan" and "Control of Illicit Drug Trafficking" in accordance with article 2 of Decree 623/96 (Honorable Congress of the Argentine Nation, 1989). This plan should contribute to the development of policies and the planning of national strategies for the prevention, training, assistance, and control of the abuse and illicit trafficking of psychoactive substances, and must ensure compliance with national and international legislation on the matter.

Public policies on addictions, in the last decade, are characterized by a poor healthcare response, an absolute absence of preventive strategies (with isolated exceptions in some provinces of the country) and a great disarticulation between the different public organizations that have specific jurisdiction and budgets for the theme. Currently, in the Ministries of Education, Health, Labor, and Justice, there are areas linked to the problem of addictions, but they generally function in a disjointed manner and often overlap. SEDRONAR fails to coordinate and articulate these areas at the national level. For this reason, it is essential to strengthen the articulating and coordinating role of SEDRONAR in the definition and consensus of a National Drug Plan for the country. We can trace the main legislative milestones on the issue of drugs in Argentina, since the possession of drugs for personal consumption is not a crime starting in 1968. As a result of a reform of the Penal Code, the penalties for trafficking are aggravated, but Law 19,567 excludes possession for personal use and mandatory confinement from criminal sanctions. In the mid-1970s, Law 20,771 was passed, punishing the possession of narcotics with imprisonment of one to six years, even when they were intended for personal use. In this context, already in the midst of the military dictatorship, the Supreme Court of Justice, in the "Colavini ruling," ratified the two-year prison sentence against Ariel Colavini, who had been found with two marijuana cigarettes.

In 1986, the Bazterrica ruling occurred, whose name refers to the surname of the guitarist of the historic Argentine rock group "Los Abuelos de la Nada," who was arrested for having drugs. In this ruling, the Supreme Court of Justice declares the unconstitutionality of article 6 of Law 20,771, which penalized the possession of drugs for personal use; the ruling was based on article 19 of the National Constitution: "The private actions of men that in no way offend public order and morality or harm a third party, are reserved only to God and exempt from the authority of the magistrates." Three years later, possession was punished (Law 23,737) with imprisonment from one month to two years and the Programming Secretariat for the Prevention of Drug Addiction and the Fight against Drug Trafficking (SEDRONAR) was created. Law 23,737 (Argentine Legal Information System, 2009), voted unanimously, sanctioned on September 21, 1989, includes the prevention and punishment of crimes linked to production, marketing, transportation, consumption, possession, etc. of narcotics. This law stands out for its rigorous penalties for drug distributors, the criminalization of those who organize and finance illicit trafficking, and a system of curative security and educational security.

In 2005, Law 26,052 allows the justice of each province and the Autonomous City of Buenos Aires to assume the investigation of minor crimes (possession and small trafficking of Law 23,737, originally attributed to the federal justice). But perhaps the most significant and controversial ruling in recent years is the so-called Arriola ruling (Milanese, 2021), which in August 2009 declared the unconstitutionality of the second paragraph of article 14 of Law 23,737, which represses the possession of substances psychoactive for personal consumption. According to the Supreme Court of Justice, the unconstitutionality of the article is applicable to those cases of possession of narcotics for personal consumption that do not affect the rights or property of third parties.

The main argument used in said ruling is that the rule that penalizes the possession of psychoactive substances for personal consumption, to the extent that it affects people's private sphere, affects the right to privacy protected by constitutional norms; not only article 19 of the National Constitution, but other international human rights instruments, incorporated after the constitutional reform of 1994. In this regard, the ruling indicates: "Possession of drugs for one's own consumption, by itself, does not offer any evidence to affirm that the accused carried out something more than a private action, that is, that they offended public morality or the rights of third parties." In that same year (2009), a group of representatives of the judiciary declared coercive treatments unconstitutional, opening the current debate on "decriminalization." (6)

Community Prevention and Risk and Harm Reduction Strategies

According to the United Nations, only 10% of problem drug users ask for help (Milanese, 2023). For this reason, community strategies are of great value for a comprehensive health system, especially if our objectives are to facilitate accessibility and reach the most vulnerable population groups in a comprehensive way.

"Community treatment" is a strategy that was born with the developments of the ECO2 model and network theories in Mexico at the end of the 1990s, and spread throughout Latin America (Machín, 2023). Currently, almost 200 civil society organizations develop treatment and evaluation strategies for cases and networks in the community in association with the Governments of Mexico, Colombia, Brazil, Peru, Uruguay, Chile, and the Autonomous City of Buenos Aires.

The ECO2 model was built from some essential elements, as a play on words: Epistemology of Complexity (ECO), Ethics and Community (ECO), therefore, ECO2. In the ECO2 model, elements are taken up that range from Mandelbrot's fractal geometry to Morin's complex thinking, passing through Wiener's cybernetics, Bateson's and Von Foerster's cybernetics, nonlinear dynamics, Haken's synergetics, Hofsdater recursion, Gell-Man adaptive complex systems, network theories, etc. (Machin, 2023). The reference "Ethics and Community" points to basic options in the intervention: respect for the dignity of people and communities, therefore, the requirement to seek to limit and counteract the phenomena of exclusion and social suffering in a professional manner, that is, that criteria of deontology, effectiveness, efficiency, and quality are satisfied. It also implies recognition and reflection by those of us who intervene, of our own motivations, limitations, errors, and the need for constant evaluation and supervision (Mansilla, 2015).

Currently, "community treatment" has instruments for monitoring and evaluating cases and changes in the community (Kornblit, Camarotti and Di Leo, 2011).

Harm reduction is one of the latest ideas in the field of treatment, heralding a paradigm shift in the way we approach problematic drug and alcohol use. Harm reduction rejects the idea that abstinence is the "only" acceptable goal for all problem users (Brasesco and Canay, 2011).

Available statistics demonstrate the need to implement a harm reduction response, in parallel and more pragmatically, to substance use disorders for the significant percentage of people who are unable to meet their own goals of treatments that are based on abstinence. If the knowledge acquired about problematic patterns of drug use is to be effectively applied in the context of prevention, treatment, and harm reduction, clear distinctions must be made between different patterns of use and between dangerousness and risk, the risks associated with the different substances that are available in licit and illicit markets.

The situation described is the starting point for the formation of local and national coalitions that demand the development of broader, more comprehensive, and effective initiatives in matters of public health, social progress, and the administration of justice within the communities. A growing group of local governments, non-governmental organizations, and entrepreneurs echo this call by demonstrating a greater commitment to achieve broader citizen participation in the implementation of this new approach and to contribute to the success of the initiatives and proposed community initiatives (Miguez, 2008). These include, for example, training of people from the communities themselves in prevention and treatment of problem drug users, harm reduction programs and education programs focused on youth, and recreational and sports activities that allow socially excluded citizens to belong to a team and not to a gang. Greater community proximity also allows for a greater flow of information that allows community members to know who needs help at any given time.

Like many structural changes, this new approach begins only gradually and becomes stronger over time. Of course, some countries and some communities advance faster than others (Brasesco and Canay, 2011; Miguez, 2008).

National Prevention Strategy

Until 2016, Argentina had not had a strategic prevention plan at the national level, which contemplated universal prevention focused on increasing the perception of risk of substance consumption, based on epidemiological studies and social representations, and much less guidelines for selective and indicated prevention at local levels.

It was expected that a national prevention plan would be based on scientific evidence and would have monitoring and evaluation indicators. Also, it was the product of dialogue and consensus between the different actors involved, including user associations. But this did not happen like that.

In 2016, the National Directorate for the Prevention of Addictions developed the National Prevention Plan as part of the SEDRONAR National Drug Plan, whose objective was aimed at having a governing framework at the national level that would guide and promote public policies on addiction prevention of the consumption of psychoactive substances, respecting criteria of accessibility, social inclusion, and human rights. Likewise, this plan saw as a perspective for action, the multicausality, and complexity of the issue in question, emphasizing the multiplicity of factors to be taken into account and the relational nature of consumption situations, proposing a comprehensive preventive approach with initiatives that range from childhood to adulthood, acting with special emphasis on adolescence and its different age stages (Brasesco and Canay, 2011; Clari, 2013; Míguez, 2001).

As a primary objective, the National Directorate for the Prevention of Addictions (DPA), proposed to design, implement, and monitor preventive public policies aimed at reducing the demand for the consumption of psychoactive substances based on universal strategies (aimed at the entire population), selective (directed at population sectors with increased risk), and indicated (focused on groups with problematic consumption). This was done in coordination with national, provincial, municipal, regional, and international organizations, in order to contribute to the comprehensive health and inclusion of the population (Míguez, 2007; SEDRONAR. 2018).

For the creation of the National Prevention Plan, the DPA took into consideration recommendations from international organizations (WHO, UN, CICAD, COPOLAD), epidemiological data on substance consumption at the national, regional, and local level generated by the Argentine Drug Observatory, OAD, and other sources (Schleimer et al., 2019; Miguez, Fernandez and Mansilla, 2010), and experiences with the implementation of preventive programs at each of the three aforementioned levels. The Plan organized the strategy into six areas of intervention: educational, contexts of confinement, work, art, sports, and nightlife.

The design of the goals in each of the six areas contemplated that SEDRONAR was not a direct executor, but rather that it should articulate its policies in the field of prevention with various governmental and non-governmental entities.[4] This articulation has been failed from the beginning, presenting a history of successive disagreements and overlaps between ministerial programs and preventive actions, of SEDRONAR, of the provinces, of the municipalities, and of the NGOs present in the Argentine Republic.

[4] National ministries with interference in the areas of prevention, such as the Ministry of Education and Sports, Ministry of Security, Ministry of Justice and Human Rights, Ministry of Health, Ministry of Social Development, and Public Prosecutor's Office; Argentine provinces, through the representatives in COFEDRO, with the respective provincial ministries; network of municipalities that have adhered to the Municipalities in Action plan; network of territorial devices of SEDRONAR and community NGOs.

Prevention in the Educational Field

Regarding the history of prevention in this area, in Argentina it has a long history. Already in 1985, the Coordinating Commission for the Control of Drug Trafficking and Drug Abuse prioritized the educational perspective of the problem of substance consumption. In that year, the non-governmental sector (Fundación Convivir) began a teacher training program in the City of Buenos Aires. From this moment on, several provinces began preventive work in the educational field, implementing actions with their own budget and guaranteeing a certain continuity over time: Buenos Aires, Jujuy, Mendoza, Chubut, Entre Ríos, La Pampa, Tucumán, Córdoba, and the Autonomous City of Buenos Aires.

Some years later, in 2007, SEDRONAR began the implementation in schools throughout the national territory of a universal prevention program whose structure was based on the Chilean Program "I want to be" (Álvarez, 2011; Raiden, 2012; Ministry of Education, 2009). For its part, two years later, the Ministry of Education began to distribute materials on protective and risk factors for substance use in public and private schools (Clari, 2013; Míguez, 2001).

Since the creation of the educational field with its own coordination in 2016, SEDRONAR assigned to said field the mission of designing, implementing, monitoring, and evaluating preventive strategies in areas of formal and non-formal education throughout the national territory. This occurred under the general guidelines of the National Directorate for the Prevention of Addictions, in inter-ministerial and inter-sectoral coordination, weaving intra- and inter-institutional networks, generating comprehensive actions for universal, selective, and indicated prevention of psychoactive substance consumption. The functions in charge of this coordination at the national level were to design preventive strategies for educational communities; monitor the development of preventive initiatives in formal and non-formal educational settings; design and implement training projects for representatives of the provincial networks in the areas of education and addictions in prevention of psychoactive substance consumption in educational settings; and develop theoretical-methodological materials on prevention for the entire educational community at all levels and modalities.

The fulfillment of these functions required articulation and agreements with various institutional bodies[5] in order to reach both direct recipients (13 million students/60,000 educational units/1 million active teachers) and indirect recipients (general, local, regional, provincial, national community).

Three strategies were organized for the implementation of the policies. The first was universal prevention, for which a theoretical-pedagogical proposal was generated in curricular guidelines, promoting certain learning for teaching drug

[5] Other areas of SEDRONAR, Ministry of Education and Sports of the Nation, NGOs, CABA, Provinces, COFEDRO delegates, Municipalities, and territorial devices; Interministerial Table of the National Council for the Coordination of Social Policies; Permanent table SEDRONAR-Ministry of Education and Sports of the Nation; Agreements with universities.

prevention during compulsory schooling. Along these lines, two printed and virtual products were produced to support the aforementioned strategies, which were distributed in all provinces of Argentine territory: Care in Games—Initial Level, and Care in Games—Primary Level.

Comprehensive preventive projects were also proposed as part of a set of theoretical-methodological mediations offered to the educational community, with the intention of accompanying training and institutional processes regarding drug prevention. Specifically, teaching training was offered for different educational levels and modalities, curricular and seminar proposals were developed for tertiary levels and universities, and prevention communication pieces in the educational field were designed, developed, and disseminated. It should be noted that this was the first time that preventive work was systematically addressed in Argentina with tertiary levels of education and universities. The proposal was quickly approved by the Federal Council of Education in 2016, in coordination with the Undersecretary of Educational Policies of the Ministry of Education and Sports.

A selective prevention proposal was also made through the design of a training project for provincial, municipal, and NGO leaders, for the implementation of preventive-educational proposals, as well as an intervention proposal was designed and developed in schools with situations of increased risk, through the generation of proximity with easily accessible community devices, called ESTAR in Prevention.

Finally, work was carried out at the level of indicated prevention, supported by a guidance guide for intervention in situations of problematic substance use at school, and preventive care networking was developed. The project also included the development of six products (delivered to schools in virtual and printed form) to support the aforementioned strategies, which were distributed in all provinces of Argentine territory: Orientation for Guidelines (theoretical-methodological guidelines for addressing the Curricular Guidelines for the Prevention of Addictions); Comprehensive Preventive Projects: Theoretical-Methodological Mediations for Educational Communities; Being in Prevention: Territorial Space for the Articulation of Networks in Prevention and Orientation for Intervention (guidance guide for intervention in situations of problematic substance use at school).

The interventions were evaluated through three instances: first, a baseline was generated that preceded the implementation of the strategies. An analysis was carried out of the situation in which the different preventive work groups found themselves in relation to the issues to be carried out within the framework of the projects, as well as the perceptions and status of the target population in relation to problematic consumption. The social representations of the problem, the knowledge of the curricular guidelines, the articulations with other organizations and health services, and the interventions that were being carried out in response to consumption situations were analyzed.

In the second instance, a process evaluation was carried out where the application of the intervention carried out by the Educational Prevention (PAE) technical team and the reactions of the participants were assessed to measure the quality of the application of the intervention, that is, the way in which they perceived the intervention and its quality. The evaluation was carried out through a survey that evaluated the impact of the intervention.

In the third instance, an evaluation of results was carried out; the specific effects of the intervention were analyzed, such as partial or total fulfillment of the planned objectives.

The ESTAR in Prevention program was developed in 20 schools in four provinces of the country (Jujuy, Catamarca, San Juan, Santiago del Estero). Regarding the process evaluation, it was carried out in 86 schools, information that was included in the process evaluation report. The evaluators were teachers, references, students, family members, and managers of the educational communities where the program was implemented. The evaluation of results was not completed since the new government that took office at the end of 2019 decided not to continue the program.

Prevention in Confinement Contexts

According to the latest United Nations report on drug consumption in Latin American penitentiaries (United Nations, 2024), people deprived of their liberty are mostly men, of which 43.7% are between 25 and 34 years. The younger incarcerated population shows lower educational levels among those up to 24 years of age.

The population deprived of liberty generally begins using psychoactive substances at a younger age than the average of the general population (18 to 65 years old) who has ever used drugs (SEDRONAR, 2019).

In Argentina, the lifetime prevalence of drug consumption in the incarcerated population is 64%. The most consumed drug is marijuana with a prevalence of 56%, followed by cocaine with 49%. In third place, and with very similar prevalence, is the consumption of hallucinogens, paste base, and ecstasy. In all cases, except for the consumption of base paste or paco, drug consumption is considerably higher in the male prison population (United Nations, 2010).

At the international level there is no doubt that intervention programs with populations deprived of liberty must be part of public policy. Most successful interventions aim, first of all, to prevent drug use in vulnerable young people or offenders, especially early onset and escalation to highly addictive drugs; and at the same time, they aim to work on reducing consumption and treatment within penitentiary institutions (Penitentiary Prosecutor's Office of the Nation, 2020).

In 2016, SEDRONAR created the area of prevention of consumption in contexts of confinement with its own coordination, with the mission of designing, implementing, and monitoring preventive strategies in the context of confinement throughout the national territory.[6]

---

[6] It should be noted that the base, process, and result evaluations of the preventive programs designed and implemented in 2016 that are cited were published on the website of the Argentine

The inter-ministerial and inter-sectoral articulation included national, provincial, municipal, and civil society organizations, linked to prevention in contexts of confinement; design and implement training projects for representatives of provincial networks in the area of confinement contexts; and inter-institutionally articulate the design and implementation of interdisciplinary devices and teams aimed at addressing problematic substance use in confinement contexts.[7] This articulation made it possible to reach a target population consisting of the population deprived of liberty throughout the country, consisting of 65.500 inmates (55,000 provincial and 10,500 federal), penitentiary personnel (total 52,000: 11,000 federal, 21,000 Buenos Aires and with an estimate of 20,000 penitentiaries in the rest of the country).

Regarding universal prevention strategies, federal and provincial actors from confinement contexts were trained, as well as key actors from institutions for minors in conflict with criminal law and actors from the justice system, Social Readaptation Program and Boards of Released Persons. And theoretical methodological contents were developed for the first time in the curricular program of the Officer and Non-Commissioned Officer Schools, in coordination with the Federal Penitentiary Service and the Provincial Penitentiary Services. These contents especially contemplated the analysis of the gender perspective, in order to design and implement responses that are appropriate to the life situation of women in contexts of confinement. As a result of the process evaluation in 2018, it turned out that five provincial and federal trainings had been carried out and, in 2017, 12 provincial and 12 federal trainings.

In turn, within the framework of selective prevention strategies, pilot tests of application of the community treatment methodology were implemented, with the consequent preparation of a registration document that acted as a process evaluation.

And, finally, the indicated prevention strategy contemplated the creation of a guide of intervention guidelines in situations of problematic substance use and an assembly of care reference routes was generated, in cases of established consumption that demand a specific methodology. Without a doubt, the indicated prevention strategy was an extremely novel contribution to public policy in confinement contexts.

Regarding the evaluation in this area, it is worth highlighting what was done in the Interinstitutional Program for Social Integration, Federal Complex II of Marcos Paz with young and adult inmates. Here, indicators were developed to evaluate the results of the strategies to address the vulnerability of young people in coordination with different ministries and NGOs. It should be noted that, to achieve the expected results, a group device was built to address problematic consumption and the

Drug Observatory of Sedronar until the end of December 2019. As of on that date, said publications were removed from the aforementioned page.

[7] Ministry of Justice and Human Rights of the Nation, Ministry of Security of the Nation, Public Prosecutor's Office, and provincial Ministries of Justice and Security. In coordination and agreements with other areas of SEDRONAR, NGOs, CABA, Provinces, COFEDRO delegates, territorial devices, and other actors involved in the context of confinement.

formation of links and the implementation of accompanying actions in the transition from confinement to the free environment were systematically promoted.

A process evaluation was also carried out in the Juvenile Criminal Responsibility Centers of the Province of Buenos Aires[8] of the formation of devices for a comprehensive approach to problematic use of psychoactive substances in four Juvenile Criminal Responsibility Centers. To this end, evaluation instruments were generated such as a registry of attendees, an assessment model for the day, an observation guide, and a monitoring record model. And finally, training sessions were held for officers and non-commissioned officers of the Federal Penitentiary Service, at the end of which a survey was administered to 300 participants to evaluate the quality of the training received. The results indicated high levels of compliance with the content worked on and the quality of the trainers.

Prevention in the Workplace

The impact of the consumption of these substances in the workplace is also very important, both in the health of the worker as well as in the activities of the organization to which it belongs. When consumption becomes problematic, it also generates costs for the organization, since more absences may occur, productivity may decrease, the risk of work accidents may increase, and interpersonal ties may deteriorate. Therefore, it is a priority to achieve and maintain optimal standards in terms of work with adequate levels of physical, mental, and social health of workers in accordance with International Labor Organization (ILO) standards. In 2017 in Argentina there were 18,237,290 people of working age between 16 and 65 years old residing in agglomerations of 80,000 or more inhabitants of the country and the 3% of this population (equivalent to around 570,000 workers) would be, according to the OAS-CICAD, affected by the consumption of psychoactive substances. In this population, according to the 2017 national study of psychoactive substance consumption in Argentina (OAD/SEDRONAR), 83% of the working-active population surveyed declared that alcohol and drug consumption at work is quite a problem (or very) important, and it also turned out that among co-workers, 31% of men and around 13% of women had excessive consumption of alcohol and/or other drugs (SEDRONAR, 2017).

Regarding measures for the prevention and assistance of substance use in the workplace, 25.5% of current workers stated that their work has some regulation that controls the use of alcohol or drugs among their employees and 18.2% received some type of information related to the prevention and consumption of drugs and/or alcohol, but only 9.6% stated that in their work there is some type of preventive/assistance program for employees with problems related to these issues (SEDRONAR, 2017).

---

[8] Municipalities of Merlo, Malvinas Argentina, Almafuerte, and Carlos Ibarra.

Data from the 2017 study put on the public agenda the need to deploy a national policy aimed at preventing or minimizing occupational risks derived from the consumption of these substances, with prevention and support programs that provide basic reference information and guide the care approach for affected workers. That is to say, the stated need to implement a substance use prevention program in the workplace was confirmed to design, implement, and monitor preventive strategies throughout the national territory, with inter-ministerial and inter-sectoral coordination, to generate comprehensive prevention actions for universal, selective, and indicated consumption of psychoactive substances.

The design of the national prevention plan in the workplace was, without a doubt, somewhat "pretentious," from the moment it included the design of universal, selective, and indicated preventive strategies, for which agreements had to be made with public spheres, national, provincial, and municipal and with companies,[9] at the same time that training proposals had to be designed for different actors in the workplace, for the implementation of prevention strategies, survey, and monitor preventive proposals and design theoretical and methodological prevention material in this area.

Basically, the plan was developed through two programs: (1) "Promoting healthy work spaces" and (2) "Good practices." The first aimed at helping to incorporate a quality of life model at work, with the vision of changing the social scenario and the mission of promoting new work and life habits and a preventive and healthy organizational culture. For this purpose, preventive promoter groups and change agents were formed in the workplace, with technical advice for the development of the preventive policy and an action plan, and advice for the development of preventive material to raise workers' awareness about the consequences of the consumption of psychoactive substances for personal, family, and work life. The program was implemented in unions/guilds and non-formal work spaces in contexts of extreme vulnerability, through meeting spaces for union and union delegates. To this end, intensive training seminars on prevention of problematic consumption were held, from a gender and human rights perspective, in person and e-learning. An evaluation of the process and results of the program was carried out.

Regarding the second program stated, "Good Practices," it focused on encouraging the exchange and development of actions and good practices such as the code of conduct and annual training actions, which promoted the implementation of a preventive culture in the workplace. At this point, the Federal Drug Council, CODEFRO, played a fundamental role in facilitating its socialization and visualization through forums, favoring the exchange of successful experiences in order to replicate them in other workplaces. In addition to the implementation of the regional forums of good practices, a national publication of good preventive practices in workplaces was prepared and an ad hoc "Certification of good practices" program was generated.

[9] The signing of the agreement was complex and involved serious delays that delayed the start of the program for several months.

The implementation of the prevention plan in the workplace reached 31 companies, 28 unions, 2 NGOs, 19 government entities, and 16 municipalities in the province of La Pampa at the national level.

Prevention in Nighttime

The 2016 prevention plan understood the need for public policies to address the expressions of nightlife and its associated risks. A specific coordination was created for the area of "nighttime," in order to develop specific actions to raise awareness of risk and care in contexts of nighttime, which included the design of specific audiovisual material, as well as brochure design and provision of supplies for risk mitigation in recreational contexts and mass events. To this end, a series of agreements on guidelines and regulations were reached with the business sector and those involved in the organization of mass events were trained in prevention and detection of risky consumption. In addition, basic emergency care conditions were created in contexts at night, established in coordination with the Ministry of Health, working in coordination with the Early Warning System (SAT) for new drugs for the continuous registration of new substances and new drugs consumption patterns within the framework of the Argentine Drug Observatory.

For the evaluation of the interventions, an instrument was developed of the interventions carried out by SEDRONAR in different mass events, in order to account for the characteristics of the event and the profile of those attending. In turn, another instrument was used to systematize information on resources allocated to prevention in terms of materials and assigned personnel, quantification of preventive actions, people assisted and referred for problems associated with consumption and main consumption modalities detected. The prevention plan in nighttime settings was developed in ten provinces of the national territory.

Conclusion

The complexity of the problems associated with drug consumption in Argentina has common denominators with other countries in the region (UNODC, 2021): cultural, socioeconomic, and psychological factors that are intertwined in the genesis; constant appearance of more adulterant New Psychoactive Substance (NPS); new consumption patterns; new sources of marketing (social networks); increase in acute clinical conditions related to a higher prevalence of drug consumption with a strong negative impact on health; proposals for legislative changes; and increased social tolerance to drug consumption due to changes in social representations in favor of a decrease in the perception of risk of drug consumption.

In past decades, quality decisions were not made in the prevention of the consumption of psychoactive substances based on evidence, even though it has been widely proven that the best solution will be one that is based on the best information (in quantity and quality), as well as in the best capacity for analysis and interpretation of that information.

It is expected that government agencies at their different levels (national, provincial, and municipal) clearly identify the problems associated with consumption and carry out good situational diagnoses, which precede decision-making regarding carrying out selective, specific, or non-specific interventions in the territories. In this way, it will be possible to carry out effective preventive interventions in the change of the situation, within the framework of systematic process monitoring and evaluation of the changes achieved from the determination of indicators agreed upon with the scientific community. It is urgent to incorporate evaluation under the criteria that are fundamental and necessary at the level of drug policies.

Furthermore, these preventive programs based on scientific evidence must together constitute an integrated system within the federal system. To achieve this, it is urgent to de-ideologize the discussion on drug policies, strengthen the institutions in charge of said policies, identify problems associated with drug consumption, its determinants and vulnerabilities, acting on the determinants (long term) and addressing the consequences (short term).

In summary, Argentina needs public policies that act in strong states and institutions, with sustained objectives and actions that can be evaluated in the long term, rather than political reactions to immediate problems. They must be based on individuals, on respect for human rights, with a balanced and multidimensional comprehensive plan approved legislatively, with a public health focus, and that lasts over time beyond the change of political administrations.

References

Álvarez, D. (2011) Evaluación del Programa de Prevención Integral sobre el Uso Indebido de Drogas en el Ámbito Educativo "Quiero Ser". Recuperado de http://www.observatorio.gov.ar/investigaciones/Evaluacion_Programa_Quiero_Ser.pdf

Archivo General de la Nación Argentina (2024). Unidad documental compuesta 3737.34 – Comisión Nacional de Toxicomanía y Narcóticos. Recuperado de Comisión Nacional de Toxicomanía y Narcóticos – Archivo General de la Nación (mininterior.gob.ar)

Brasesco, V., & Canay, R. (2011) Sentido social en la investigación epidemiológica en adicciones. *Observatorio Social, (32)*, 12-13.

Camarotti, A. C., & Güelman, M. (2018). Historia de los tratamientos para los consumos de drogas.

Canay, R., & Brasesco, M. V. (2014). Adicciones. Consumo de drogas legales e ilegales. *Edicon. Fondo Editorial Consejo. Consejo Profesional de Ciencias Económicas de la Ciudad Autónoma de Buenos Aires.*

Centro de Referencia Nacional en Salud Mental (s.f.). Recuperado de www.argentina.gob.ar/salud/hospitalbonaparte/institucional/historia

CICAD (2010). Estrategia Hemisférica sobre Drogas. Recuperado de https://www.suin-juriscol.gov.co/derechos/Estrategia-esp.pdf

Clari, P. L. (2013). Prevención de adicciones: el docente como educador en la promoción de habilidades preventivas en adolescentes que cursan el ciclo orientado. Recuperado de https://repositorio.uca.edu.ar/bitstream/123456789/567/1/doc.pdf

Gil, M. (2022). Los abordajes de la SEDRONAR en la República Argentina (1989-2019): Hacia una historización de políticas públicas sobre consumo problemático de sustancias desde una perspectiva antropológica relacional.
Honorable Congreso de la Nación Argentina (1989). Ley 23737 Modificación al Código Penal. Recuperado de www.argentina.gob.ar/normativa/nacional/ley-23737-138
Honorable Congreso de la Nación Argentina (2010). Ley 26.657. Derecho a la Protección de la Salud Mental. Disposiciones complementarias. Derógase la Ley N° 22.914. Recuperado de www.argentina.gob.ar/normativa/nacional/ley-26657-175977
Instituto Nacional de Estadística y Censo de Argentina (2024). Recuperado de www.indec.gob.ar
Kornblit, A. L., Camarotti, A. C., & Di Leo, P. F. (2011). Prevención del consumo problemático de drogas: Módulo 1 La construcción social de la problemática de las drogas. Recuperado de https://infanciayjuventudsc.wordpress.com/wp-content/uploads/2011/05/1-construccic3b3n-social-de-la-problemc3a1tica-de-las-drogas2.pdf
Machín, J. (2023). La prevención de las farmacodependencias en el Modelo Eco2. Recuperado de https://liberaddictus.org/Pdf/0799-75.pdf
Mansilla, J. C. (2015). Apuntes Históricos de la Política Pública en Consumo de Drogas de Argentina. Blog personal. Recuperado de http://juanenlinea.blogspot.com.ar/2015/05/apuntes-historicos-de-la-politica.html
Milanese, E. (2021). Un abordaje a la reducción del daño. Proceso de formación con equipos de la Organización Samaritanos de la Calle, Cali, Colombia 2021-2022. Recuperado de www.academia.edu/95365961/Efrem_Milanese_Un_abordaje_a_la_reducción_del_daño_septiembre_2021
Milanese, E. (2023). Tratamiento Comunitario. Manual de trabajo Eco2. Drogas y exclusión grave. *Síntesis*. Recuperado de www.academia.edu/36204845/Tratamiento_Comunitario_Manual_de_Trabajo_Tercera_Edición_2016
Miguez, H. (2008). Estilos de vida y emocionalidad producida en adicciones. Modernidad, Tecnología y síntomas contemporáneos. AASM. *Reguillo*.
Míguez, H. A. (2001). Fundamento para una tarea preventiva. In *Trabajo presentado en el III Congreso Internacional sobre adicciones del programa Cambio. Abstract del congreso. Córdoba*. Recuperado de www.hugomiguez.com.ar/prev1.pdf
Míguez, H. A. (2007). Abuso de sustancias psicoactivas: sobre la prevención. *Acta Psiquiátrica y Psicológica de América Latina*, *53*(3), 157.
Miguez, H., Fernandez, R., & Mansilla, J. C. (2010). Estudio exploratorio sobre el imaginario de la nocturnidad, la alcoholización y la diversión juvenil. *Córdoba: Secretaría de Coordinación en Prevención y Asistencia de las Adicciones*.
Ministerio de Educación (2009). El Programa Nacional de Educación y Prevención Sobre las Adicciones y el Consumo Indebido de Drogas. http://portal.educacion.gov.ar/files/2013/10/adiccion_prevencion.pdf
Ministerio de Justicia (2016). Relatoría del encuentro y del taller sobre el futuro del proceso de regionalización de la política de drogas en Colombia. Tercer Encuentro Nacional de Regionalización de la Política de Drogas Bogotá, 27 y 28 de octubre de 2016. Recuperado de www.minjusticia.gov.co/programas-co/ODC/Documents/Territorios/relatoria_tercer_encuentro_regional_2016.pdf
Ministerio de Salud (s.f.). Acerca del Observatorio Argentino de Drogas. Recuperado de www.argentina.gob.ar/sedronar/observatorio-argentino-de-drogas/acerca
Naciones Unidas (2010). Consumo de Drogas en Población Privada de Libertad y la relación entre Droga y Delito. Cuarto Informe Conjunto. Sistema Subregional de Información e Investigación sobre Drogas en Argentina, Bolivia, Chile, Colombia, Ecuador, Perú y Uruguay. Recuperado de www.argentina.gob.ar/sites/default/files/2020/10/unodc_2010._consumo_de_drogas_en_poblacion_privada_de_la_libertad_y_la_relacion_entre_delito_y_droga_cuarto_informe_conjunto.pdf
Naciones Unidas (2024). Informe Mundial sobre las Drogas 2024 de UNODC: los daños del problema mundial de las drogas siguen aumentando en medio de la expansión del consumo y los mercados de drogas. Recuperado de www.unodc.org/unodc/es/press/releases/2024/June/unodc-world-drug-report-2024_-harms-of-world-drug-problem-continue-to-mount-amid-expansions-in-drug-use-and-markets.html

Parga, J. (2016). "Salir del bardo": Etnografía de las políticas públicas de abordaje del consumo de sustancias en la provincia de Buenos Aires (1993-2011).
Poder Ejecutivo Nacional (P.E.N.) (1996). Prevención de la drogadicción y la lucha contra el narcotráfico Decreto 623/96. Recuperado de www.argentina.gob.ar/normativa/nacional/decreto-623-1996-37570
Procuración Penitenciaria de la Nación (2020). Cárcel y consumos problemáticos. Recuperado de https://www.ppn.gov.ar/pdf/ejestematicos/SaludMental/Disertaciones-Consumo-problematico-y-carceles.pdf
Raiden, M. (2012). *Razón, verdad y experiencia en Prevención de Adicciones: Análisis de la retórica preventiva del Programa Nacional* "Quiero Ser". (Master's thesis, Buenos Aires: FLACSO. Sede Académica Argentina).
Schleimer, J. P., Rivera-Aguirre, A. E., Castillo-Carniglia, A., Laqueur, H. S., Rudolph, K. E., Suárez, H., et al. (2019). Investigating how perceived risk and availability of marijuana relate to marijuana use among adolescents in Argentina, Chile, and Uruguay over time. *Drug and alcohol dependence*, *201*, 115-126.
SEDRONAR (2017). Consumo de Sustancias Psicoactivas y Mercado laboral. Estudio Nacional en Población de 12 a 65 Años Sobre Consumo de Sustancias Psicoactivas. Recuperado de https://www.argentina.gob.ar/sites/default/files/2020/10/oad_2017._consumo_de_sustancias_psicoactivas_y_mercado_laboral_estudio_nacional_en_poblacion_de_12_a_65_anos.pdf
SEDRONAR (2018). Resumen informe de evaluación: Conformación de dispositivos de abordaje integral en red de los consumos problemáticos de sustancias psicoactivas en Centros de Responsabilidad Penal Juvenil de la Provincia de Buenos Aires, Argentina, 2017-2018. Recuperado de https://www.argentina.gob.ar/sites/default/files/2020/11/oad_2019._conformacion_de_dispositivos_de_abordaje_de_los_consumos_problematicos_en_centros_de_resp._penal_juvenil.pdf
SEDRONAR (2019). Conformación de dispositivos de abordaje integral en red de los consumos problemáticos de sustancias psicoactivas en Centros de Responsabilidad Penal Juvenil de la Provincia de Buenos Aires. ARGENTINA, 2017 – 2018. Recuperado de www.argentina.gob.ar/sites/default/files/2020/10/oad_2019._conformacion_de_dispositivos_de_abordaje_de_los_consumos_problematicos_en_centros_de_resp._penal_juvenil.pdf
Sistema Argentino de Información Jurídica (SAIJ) (2009). Recurso de hecho causa n° 9080. Recuperado de SAIJ – Arriola, Sebastián y otros s/ RECURSO DE HECHO causa n° 9080
UNODC (2013). Los tratados de fiscalización internacional de drogas. Recuperado de www.argentina.gob.ar/sites/default/files/the_international_drug_control_conventions_s.pdf
UNODC (2021). Drogas sintéticas y Nuevas sustancias psicoactivas en América Latina y el Caribe 2021. Recuperado de https://www.unodc.org/documents/scientific/21-02921_LAC_drug_assessment_S_ebook.pdf
Wrobel, G. (2006). Programas y políticas de estado en materia de prevención de consumo de sustancias psicoactivas en Argentina, América y Europa. Estado de situación mundial. Recuperado de http://www.observatorio.gov.ar/especificos/informesinternacionales/2006_OEI05_Politicasde_Prevencion_de_Drogas_en_el_Mundo.pdf

Roberto Canay Ph.D., Universidad del Salvador, Master's degree in Community Mental Health, University of Cagliari, Italy. Specialist in community addiction treatment, University of Paraíba, Brazil; member of the Editorial Board of the scientific journal "Adiktologie" (Czech Republic); and of the Scientific Committee of the Acta Psiquiátrica y Psicológica de América Latina journal. He is currently a consultant and project coordinator for the Inter-American Drug Abuse Control Commission (CICAD) of the Organization of American States. He was Undersecretary for the Prevention and Treatment of Addictions for the Government of the Republic of Argentina.

Maria Veronica Brasesco Ph.D., Università degli Studi di Bologna, specialist in Child and Adolescent Mental Health, R. Gutierrez Children's Hospital, Buenos Aires. Undergraduate and postgraduate lecturer at the Universidad del Museo Social and Universidad del Salvador (Argentina) and at the Universidad Católica (Uruguay); researcher in Epidemiology and Issues Related to Drug Use and Other Addictive Practices.

Prevention Science in Australia

John W. Toumbourou, Bosco Rowland, Renati Solomon, Shree Solomon, Afonso Soares, Simao do Rosario, Hua-Hie Yong, Bianca Klettke, Elizabeth Clancy, Adrian Kelly, and Jacqueline Allen

J. W. Toumbourou (✉) · H.-H. Yong · B. Klettke · E. Clancy
Deakin University, School of Psychology and Centre for Social and Early Emotional Development, Geelong, VIC, Australia
e-mail: john.toumbourou@deakin.edu.au; hua.yong@deakin.edu.au; bianca.klettke@deakin.edu.au; elizabeth.clancy@deakin.edu.au

B. Rowland
Deakin University, School of Psychology and Centre for Social and Early Emotional Development, Geelong, VIC, Australia

Monash University, Richmond, VIC, Australia
e-mail: bosco.rowland@monash.edu.au

R. Solomon
Veer Wajekar College, Navi Mumbai, India
e-mail: renati.solomon@deakin.edu.au

S. Solomon
Martin Luther Christian University, Shillong, Meghalaya, India

A. Soares · S. do Rosario
Timor Leste Ministry of Education, United States Aid Organization, Dili, Timor-Leste

A. Kelly
Queensland University of Technology, Brisbane City, QLD, Australia
e-mail: a.kelly@qut.edu.au

J. Allen
Griffith University Australia, Brisbane City, QLD, Australia
e-mail: jacqueline.allen@griffith.edu.au

A. Pérez-Gómez, J. Mejía-Trujillo (eds.), *Drug Abuse Prevention*, Advances in Mental Health and Addiction, https://doi.org/10.1007/978-3-031-99621-4_2

Country Context

Australia is a continent and an island located between the Indian and South Pacific Oceans, geographically positioned both in the Southern and Eastern hemispheres of the earth. Within the United Nations (UN) groupings, Australia is classified as part of the Oceania (Pacific) countries and is grouped as near the Asian (Southern, South-Eastern, Eastern and Central Asia) countries. In 2024, the UN estimated the Australian population at 26.7 million people. The Indigenous Aboriginal and Torres Strait Islander people and nations of Australia are the traditional custodians of the land, having inhabited it for an estimated 60,000 years. In 1788 British settlers claimed Australia as a new territory of Britain, initiating ongoing experiences of violence, dispossession and cultural loss for the First Nations people. The 2021 Australian census noted 27.6% of the population were born overseas. The top five ancestries were English (33.0%), Australian (29.9%), Irish (9.5%), Scottish (8.6%) and Chinese (5.5%).

Introduction

This chapter has been written by the Inaugural Committee for the Asia-Pacific Society for Prevention Research to provide our perspective on the history and status of prevention science in Australia. We comment on the relevance of prevention advances for the regions of the Asia-Pacific where Australia is located. Our reflections are based on our discipline experience in psychology, health promotion (public health) and criminology.

In this chapter we focus on prevention research and practice in Australia. However, we also describe how Australian prevention efforts relate to broader public health challenges in the Asia-Pacific region.

Prevention in a Public Health Context

Although it can be challenging to design and implement interventions and to complete evaluation trials, there is a mounting body of social and economic evidence indicating that interventions at the level of states, municipalities, neighbourhoods, workplaces or educational institutions can improve health and social outcomes for large populations (Toumbourou et al., 2014; Vos et al., 2010). National public health systems can be conceptualised as a major universal approach to advancing health. This approach follows a staged model, such that data are first systematically collected on problems and determining influences. These data then enable the informed selection of suitable interventions that address problems and determinants. Approaches are said to be evidence-based where they make use of data from previous program evaluations and aetiological research to inform their design and to increase their potential to reduce targeted problems.

Prevention refers here to strategies or programs that avert or delay the onset of health, mental health or social problems. Prevention responses can be classified as universal where they apply to an entire population, selective where they target groups with elevated risk, and indicated where they target individuals already showing signs or symptoms of illness. This conceptualisation of prevention addresses the progression from risk factor to illness within populations (Muñoz et al., 1996).

Prevention encompasses goals not just for reducing illness, but also for reducing illness determinants. For example, Australian tobacco, alcohol and drug policies include a broad set of goals not just to reduce demand for tobacco, and hazardous alcohol and drug use, but also to reduce the supply of tobacco, alcohol and drugs, and the contexts where use results in harm (Toumbourou et al., 2018). Increasing the capacity to reduce both demand and supply is also relevant in efforts to decrease sedentary behaviour and unhealthy food consumption (Miller et al., 2013).

Prevention approaches are attractive from an economic perspective, offering the potential to reduce problems that can otherwise overburden the health systems. Within a rational public health approach, prevention priorities and targets are typically based on epidemiological estimations of the burden (or disability) associated with a specific disease. Psychologists have assisted in developing measures of disease burden in chronically ill (e.g., Browne et al., 2012) and national populations (e.g., Vos et al., 2010). All other factors being equal, it is important to ensure that the health problems that contribute the greatest share of individual, societal and economic distress receive the highest priority. On equity grounds, sub-populations such as Indigenous and socioeconomically disadvantaged populations that shoulder a disproportionate share of the health burden should also receive priority attention.

Integrating Across Multiple Domains to Prevent Health and Social Problems

An important focus in health promotion and preventative approaches involves efforts to integrate activities across multiple domains of influence. Modern health promotion approaches emphasise the importance of cultural, policy and system influences as determinants of population health outcomes (United Nations, 2016). A systems approach to prevention acknowledges the range of political and economic mechanisms operating at global, national and state levels that can impact on health issues. These include international treaties, and national and state policies and investments. Many factors at the community level mediate the impact of state and national policies. For example, numerous services and policies are coordinated and delivered by regionalised health services, local government and community health services, and through workplaces and educational institutions (Toumbourou et al., 2014).

Longitudinal Studies of Healthy Development

Longitudinal studies offer the potential to identify the developmental course and predictors of health and disease in different populations. Longitudinal studies have been increasingly used to identify the predictors of priority health problems such as alcohol (Meque et al., 2019) and tobacco use (Wellman et al., 2016). Longitudinal research highlights the potential to prevent health and social problems by ensuring optimal conditions for child and youth development and by promoting healthy lifestyle behaviour in the early years (Toumbourou, 2016).

Prevention science approaches aim to direct evidence-based investment to modify the early developmental pathways and influences that lead to later problems. Together with other disciplines, many areas of psychology have contributed to this integrated prevention science approach including: health, clinical, applied social, community and organisational psychology. Prevention can be used to deliver services and programs to reduce the incidence of health and social problems later in life, but to enable this possibility, systems for monitoring healthy child and adolescent development are required.

Researchers from our team have made important contributions to the study of healthy development across the life-course through unique cross-national comparative longitudinal studies (https://lifecourse.org.au/). Our comparative analyses have shed light on cross-national similarities and differences in youth health and social problems and modifiable influences that can be targeted in community prevention programs. These analyses have shown lower rates of youth alcohol and drug use in India relative to Australia, the USA and Europe (Rowland, Jonkman, et al., 2021), suggesting that social norms and supply regulations operating in India might have protective benefits for youth in other nations. Findings that show cross-nationally similar school and community clustering of youth health and social problems in places of disadvantage suggest that there may be common approaches to targeting of youth behavioural (Parks et al., 2020) and mental health (Lewis et al., 2017) problems. These findings provide foundations for cross-national exchange in the development of health promotion programs.

Risk and Protective Factors That Influence Health

Modifiable risk factors for cardio-vascular disease (CVD) include: smoking, high blood pressure, high body mass index (BMI) and unfavourable lipid levels (cholesterol). These factors have a cumulative impact on CVD, with similar risks for Australia/New Zealand and Asian populations (Peters et al., 2018).

Borrowing similar techniques to those used in the study of risk and protective factors for CVD, researchers have investigated risk and protective factors that influence the development of child and youth health and social problems. In the analysis of longitudinal studies, developmental risk factors are defined as independent predictors of health and/or social problems. Although protective factors are often defined as the reverse of risk factors, they are more clearly differentiated as characteristics that buffer, mediate or moderate the influence of risk factors, thereby reducing the likelihood of later problems for populations at greatest risk of poor health. Resilience researchers have identified several protective factors by studying children who have avoided adversity after being exposed to difficult childhood experiences such as parental mental illness or extreme poverty; identifying characteristics at the individual, family and community levels (Catalano & Hawkins, 1996; Haggerty & McCowan, 2018). Protective factors are described further in the text below.

To empower community action, it can be useful to identify risk and protective factors that can be modified at the community level by supporting individual, family, organisational and neighbourhood change. These factors can be differentiated from structural determinants that affect large populations and require modification through state, national and international action. As one example, at the structural level socioeconomic disadvantage is a characteristic that is consistently associated with developmental problems for children and adolescents, and is most effectively addressed through state, national and international economic actions, working in concert with community efforts (Toumbourou et al., 2007).

Community level action may be able to modify several community risk factors that influence adolescent substance use (e.g., Catalano & Hawkins, 1996; Hawkins et al., 1992) and obesity (Mathews et al., 2010) including normative expectations for behaviour and the availability of harmful substances and unhealthy food. Within the community, risk factors at the family, school and peer levels influence a range of adolescent health behaviours. For example, family and peer tobacco use are risk factors for children adopting this behaviour (Van Ryzin et al., 2012). Unhealthy food availability at school is a modifiable risk factor for student unhealthy food consumption (Yoong et al., 2016).

While greater attention is often given to identifying and targeting modifiable risk factors, it is equally important to consider those factors that promote resilience and are therefore protective. The social development strategy (SDS) emphasises the role of social bonding as an important modifiable protective factor. According to the SDS, vulnerable groups such as racial minorities and children in poverty can be protected through prosocial bonding encouraged by programs that build opportunities, skills, rewards and recognition (Haggerty & McCowan, 2018). Exposing children to programs of this type can help them to feel bonded to their community, families and schools. Community collaboration to implement programs of this type can also develop prosocial community standards and norms that are important protective factors across large populations.

Social and economic mobility patterns in Australia and other countries have increased socioeconomic differentials and led to a situation whereby children experiencing risk trajectories tend to be disproportionately clustered within disadvantaged geographic regions, communities and schools (Doery et al., 2022; Parks et al., 2020). The solution is to invest within these targeted areas to prevent the potential for an avalanching snowball of risk factors (Toumbourou et al., 2014) by building protective solutions and reducing early life risk factors. For example, by increasing support and the availability of substance use treatment to mothers in disadvantaged communities, before they conceive, it may be possible to prevent the sequence of events that can result in the cumulative escalation of risk (Catalano et al., 2012).

Synthesising Understanding of Intervention Processes and Program Logic

While behavioural and health psychology frameworks have been identified above, understanding the process and logic behind large scale, universal and multicomponent programs is a critical element in identifying effective evidence. Multicomponent interventions are necessary as the development of health behaviours are often the consequence of a variety of risk factors. Several planning frameworks have been developed to organise the evidence into a coherent and sound intervention. One popular approach organises complex ecological interventions by considering leverage points in predisposing (e.g., community attitudes, beliefs and skills relevant to desired behaviour change), reinforcing (e.g., social norms and economic factors that may support the desired behaviour change) and enabling factors (e.g., availability and accessibility of resources, or services that facilitate behaviour change) (Green & Kreuter, 2005). A similar approach is used for intervention mapping (Bartholomew Eldrigde et al., 2016).

Economic analysis is a further method that is being used to synthesise the range of evaluation evidence to reach conclusions as to which "portfolio" of investments would be most efficient in reducing the burden of disease within a population (Vos et al., 2010). To offer meaningful conclusions, economic analyses require good quality information on the aetiology of disorders and well-controlled evaluations of a range of interventions.

Structural and Macro Policy Interventions at the National/State Levels

Structural inequality and socioeconomic differentials are elevated in the Asian nations, where women receive some of the lowest share of income internationally (World Inequality Lab, 2022). These inequalities adversely impact children and adolescents and typically require national and state action to be effectively addressed. State, national and international advocacy can reduce inequalities for women (Satyen et al., 2020). Community-managed strategies to reduce inter-generational disadvantage that have evidence from the United States and Australian trials include supportive home visiting to socioeconomically disadvantaged families (Goldfeld et al., 2021, 2022) and programs to improve disadvantaged educational environments (Toumbourou et al., 2007).

Supportive home visiting programs to socioeconomically disadvantaged families (typically mothers are targeted) seek to reduce early childhood risk factors related to poor parenting and family stress, which can contribute to inter-generational disadvantage by reducing a child's potential for educational achievement and economic mobility (Goldfeld et al., 2021, 2022). Programs to improve primary school teaching and behaviour management practices have been demonstrated in the United States (Hawkins et al., 2005). Australian trials are underway (Baffsky et al., 2022) to improve early educational environments and thereby increase school success rates and disrupt the continuation of inter-generational disadvantage.

In Australia, the major structural interventions that have been proposed to prevent adolescent health priority problems are taxation reforms to reduce economic access to alcohol and tobacco and increased industry regulation to control the marketing and availability of alcohol and tobacco (Vos et al., 2010; Borland & Yong, 2018). Although similar controls have been proposed to reduce access to unhealthy foods, there have been few evaluations. While there has been success in implementing tax and regulatory reforms relevant to tobacco (Dessaix et al. 2016), recommended reforms relevant to alcohol and unhealthy food have not been implemented. Developing media and advocacy strategies and communicating evidence to align public opinion with evidence-based public health reforms can play a valuable role in preventing health and social problems (e.g., Borland & Yong, 2018; Rowland, Kremer, et al., 2021).

As relevant to health promotion, the sections that follow outline regional progress in the attainment of sections of the United Nations Sustainable Development Goals. We highlight examples of how risk factors have been identified and interventions evaluated.

Australian and Regional Trends in United Nations Sustainable Development Goals for Health

The United Nations (2016) Sustainable Development Goals (SDGs) set health targets to be achieved by all countries by 2030. Within the 17 Goals, Goal 3 set targets for "Good health and wellbeing". We examine progress on a section of the targets subsumed under Goal 3 within the United Nations regions incorporating the Asian (Southern, South-Eastern, Eastern and Central Asia) and Oceania (Pacific) countries.

SDG Target 3.1 aims to "reduce the global maternal mortality ratio to less than 70 per 100,000 live births". Progress reports (United Nations, 2020) graph impressive reductions within the region from 2000 to 2017. In Australia and the nearby island country of New Zealand, the rate of 20 maternal deaths per 100,000 births continued below the international target throughout the period examined. These reductions bring responsibilities to equitably share health system advances within the wider region where maternal deaths are improving but remain above the UN target in many countries. Progress reports (United Nations, 2020) graph from 2000 to 2017 reductions from 380 down to 150 per 100,000 live births in Central and Southern Asia; 120 down to 70 in Eastern and South-East Asia; and 220 down to 120 in Oceania, excluding Australia and New Zealand.

SDG Target 3.2 aims to "reduce neonatal mortality to at least as low as 12 per 1,000 live births and under-5 mortality to at least as low as 25 per 1,000 live births". Progress reports (United Nations, 2020) examining regional reductions from 2000 to 2018 show Australia and New Zealand under the international target at below 10 throughout the period. However, while progress is evident, under-5 mortality remains above the UN target in many neighbouring countries. From 2000 to 2018 regional reductions were observed from 95 down to 45 deaths per 1000 under 5s in Central and Southern Asia; 45 down to 15 in Eastern and South-East Asia; and 65 down to 50 in Oceania, excluding Australia and New Zealand.

To reduce maternal and child mortality, it is important to reduce modifiable risk factors such as family violence. Fulu et al. (2017) have assessed risk factors and note reciprocal relationships between child maltreatment, harsh discipline and violence against women in the Asia and Pacific region. An Australian psychology team led by Dr Lata Satyen (Satyen et al., 2020) reviewed the evidence for programs to reduce violence against women and noted several promising programs that could be implemented in the region: including advocacy for policy change and family and community health promotion.

Home visiting programs for socioeconomically disadvantaged mothers provide one example of an effective model that could be more widely implemented in the Asia-Pacific region. These programs have evidence for improving maternal and infant health in vulnerable families (University of Colorado, 2022; Washington State Institute for Public Policy, 2019). In recent decades, home visiting programs have been evaluated in Australia demonstrating health benefits for socioeconomically disadvantaged mothers and their children (Goldfeld et al., 2021, 2022).

Martin et al. (2020) reviewed evidence supporting behavioural interventions in low-and-middle-income countries (LMICs) to increase family support for maternal and child nutrition. This review concluded that behavioural interventions were both feasible and potentially effective for supporting maternal and child health in LMICs.

SDG Target 3.4 aims to "reduce by one third premature mortality from non-communicable diseases through prevention and treatment and promote mental health and well-being". Liou et al. (2020) report national differences in life expectancy and note that most countries have made similar gains at younger ages. However, in older cohorts from age 75 onwards, differences between countries become evident. Asian nations have lower life expectancies for older adults relative to high income nations, with Oceania (excluding Australia and New Zealand) having amongst the lowest life expectancy for older adults. A systematic review suggests that community level interventions can be an effective strategy for reducing CVD risk factors in LMICs (van de Vijver et al., 2012).

Australian community interventions have been demonstrated to reduce adolescent risk factors for obesity in the areas of physical activity and healthy nutrition

(Mathews et al., 2010). These interventions could be adapted and tested for their application to LMICs. The existence of inequalities in life expectancy together with evidence for effective interventions suggests directions to support efforts to encourage healthy lifestyle programs within the Asia and Oceania regions.

SDG Target 3.5 aims to "strengthen the prevention and treatment of substance abuse, including narcotic drug abuse and harmful use of alcohol". Over the past decades, Australian health psychologists have made important contributions to reducing rates of youth alcohol, tobacco and illicit drug use (Guerin & White, 2020; Toumbourou et al., 2018). Reductions in youth tobacco use can be attributed to programs and policies that reduce the demand for tobacco by adolescents and control its supply to this vulnerable group via strategies such as the dissemination of information on the harms of tobacco use (Borland and Yong, 2018) and effective family and school prevention programs (Toumbourou et al., 2018, 2019). Australian reductions in school-age alcohol use have been attributed to programs and policies that have reduced the supply of alcohol to adolescents by adults and parents (Toumbourou et al., 2018). Reductions in illicit drug use have been related to community coalition programs to encourage healthy development for children and adolescents (Toumbourou et al., 2019).

Communities That Care (CTC) is a 5-phase coalition training model that was developed by researchers from the University of Washington in the USA. Over the past two decades, members of our team supported the establishment of a not-for-profit company to adapt, evaluate and disseminate the CTC model in Australia. Through this model, local auspice agencies (e.g., Local Councils/Municipalities) appoint community co-ordinators and host CTC coalitions (Phases 1 and 2). In Phase 3 local coalitions completed community profiles that use valid child and youth surveys of preventable health and social problems and modifiable influences. This information was used to guide the selection of evidence-based prevention programs that were implemented in Phase 4, and then evaluated by repeating surveys in Phase 5.

The Australian CTC company continues to provide standardised training and technical support to guide coalitions. The Australian CTC model has been shown to be effective in preventing youth alcohol (Rowland, Kremer, et al., 2021), tobacco and cannabis use (Toumbourou et al., 2019), injury hospitalisation (Berecki-Gisolf et al., 2020) and police reported crime (Rowland et al., 2022).

SDG Target 3.6 aims to "halve the number of global deaths and injuries from road traffic accidents". Although high income nations tend to have lower death and injury from road traffic accidents than LMICs, Australia has been noted for achieving particularly low rates of road trauma. For example, Marshall (2018) reported that annual road death rates were 5.3 per 100,000 road users in Australia, which was less than half those in the United States (12.4 per 100,000). Marshall explained this to be due to more assertive Australian policies on: seat belts, driving while drug or alcohol affected, lowering vehicle speeds, safer roads and vehicles, older youth licensing ages and safer alternative transport options. Psychological and behaviour change theories have made important contributions to road safety science (Zou and Vu, 2019). In recent developments, Australia is leading strategic efforts to achieve zero road deaths through strategies that include policy development, public health messaging and safer vehicle and road design (Marshall, 2018).

In their analysis, Wismans et al. (2016) note large regional disparities in road deaths and injuries, with trends showing high and rising problems in the Asian region. These disparities suggest that prevention professionals including those in psychology and public health can play an important role by advocating health promotion measures that have been successful in Australia to equitably reduce road death and injury in the Asia-Pacific region.

SDG Target 3.A aims to "strengthen the implementation of the World Health Organization Framework Convention on Tobacco Control in all countries, as appropriate". Significant reductions in tobacco use have been achieved within the Australian school-age population (Guerin & White, 2020; Toumbourou et al., 2018) because of deliberate large-scale public health strategies aimed at reducing this behaviour and influencing factors. Strategies have included: social marketing to promote unfavourable attitudes to tobacco; economic and taxation interventions to ensure financial disincentives for purchasers; state laws that both limit the environments where it is legal to smoke and restrict access to tobacco by minors; and reductions in the prevalence of smoking among adult role models (Borland & Yong, 2018). New Zealand has also embarked on an ambitious tobacco control program, setting a target to reduce daily smoking prevalence to less than 5% by 2025 through radical measures such as allowing only sales of very low nicotine content cigarettes, drastically reducing retail outlet availability and introducing a smoke-free generation policy, all with the aim to eliminate all combustible tobacco use (Daube & Maddox, 2021; Lang & Braillon, 2022).

As tobacco use has reduced in high-income nations such as Australia and New Zealand, tobacco companies have focussed on developing new markets in LMICs. Hence, while tobacco-related deaths are declining in high-income countries, the number of annual tobacco-related deaths in LMICs is projected to increase to 6.8 million by 2030 (Mathers & Loncar, 2006). In 2020, the prevalence of tobacco use among adult males (15 years and older) was high relative to world averages (34.3%) in the WHO Southeast Asian (46.6%) and the Western Pacific regions (46.4%) (World Health Organization, 2021). Cross-national behavioural studies have compared tobacco use noting low rates for women in Asia, while harmful impacts on cardiovascular health are similar in Asian and Caucasian populations (Peters et al., 2018).

Researchers have noted new trends for youth e-cigarette use in Southeast Asian countries, partly driven by tobacco and e-cigarette company marketing tactics (Stubbs, Thomas, Pitt, & Daube, 2022). Tobacco company marketing practices that have been banned in Australia and other high-income countries are being used to attract young males to tobacco use in Southeast Asia. Research has noted the use in Cambodia of marketing practices that include tobacco sponsorships (Stubbs, 2021), promotions (Stubbs, White, Kong, & Toumbourou, 2022) and packet advertising (Stubbs, White, & Toumbourou, 2022). These findings support the need to strengthen the implementation of the WHO Framework Convention for Tobacco Control (FCTC) within the region, particularly among LMICs.

Supporting local community coalitions offers a feasible method for prevention professionals to advocate evidence-based policies. In 2015, our health psychology research team members met Mr Thomas Lopes handing out Seventh Day Adventist tobacco use prevention literature in Timor-Leste. Mr Lopes, working as an employee of the Australian charity *Many Hands* (https://manyhands.org.au/), was subsequently supported to complete health promotion units at Deakin University in Australia. Mr Lopes consulted political and regional leaders and identified agreement that the prevention of tobacco use should be given a higher priority. Mr Lopes facilitated the establishment of the Timor Leste Alliance for Tobacco Control in 2016. The Alliance has subsequently been successful in lobbying the government of Timor Leste to implement the FCTC. The first tobacco cessation programs, sales regulation and enforcement and tobacco free space programs were implemented in Timor Leste with assistance from the Alliance, guided by Deakin University health psychologists who provided advice on effective health promotion strategies. In 2022, tobacco tax reform was successfully achieved in Timor-Leste with advocacy and advice from the Alliance guided by a Deakin University report (Toumbourou et al., 2021). In 2024 the Timor Leste government has adopted UN targets to reduce non-communicable disease burden by 25% by 2030 and our prevention science team will assist this achievement.

Future Directions for Prevention Science in Australia and the Asia-Pacific Region

Australia's experience setting up a modern public health system and health research and training facilities provides an important opportunity to cooperate internationally to assist healthy development within the Asia-Pacific region. In their review, Catalano et al. (2012) identified the potential to promote the worldwide implementation of prevention science programs with the goal of reducing sexually transmissible infection, preventing harmful alcohol and tobacco use and obesity and empowering women to control their lives and fertility. The Catalano et al. (2012) review identified the requirement to address structural policies at the national/state levels and to implement effective interventions at the community, school, family and individual/peer-levels. Relevant structural policies supported by at least quasi-experimental evidence in their review included: adolescent access to contraception; taxation to reduce the economic availability of alcohol and tobacco; raising the legal age for alcohol use and purchase to 21; and graduated licensing to reduce alcohol-related harm among drivers. Effective interventions include: mentorship at the community level; school reorganisation and health curricula; parent education and family therapy; and web-based and interactive skill development interventions for individuals and peer groups (Catalano et al., 2012).

With success in managing infectious diseases and in reducing risk factors for injury, health promotion is exploring a new and broader range of options for encouraging optimal health (Toumbourou, 2016). New approaches to health are moving away from the disease model to examine positive development and wellbeing through social contribution and participation. Conceptions of thriving in Positive Youth Development suggest the possibility that the developmental interests of young people may be best served where they are encouraged and supported to provide service to others through ambitious plans such as the UN SDGs. An experimental trial randomly assigned adolescent students (n = 52, average age 15) to a weekly volunteering condition involving mentoring of elementary school students. Comparisons with control students engaged in their usual school program (n = 54) found that biological risk factors for heart disease including cholesterol and body mass index were reduced in the intervention group (Schreier et al., 2013).

Conclusion

This chapter has demonstrated that knowledge from prevention science and health promotion has made important contributions to advancing areas of human development in Australia that have relevance to the challenge in the broader Asia-Pacific region to achieve the UN SDG targets focussed for health and wellbeing. Prevention and health promotion professionals have contributed to demonstrable advances in preventative health in Australia in areas relevant to tobacco control, injury, youth alcohol and drug use and the reduction of intergenerational risk factors for poor health outcomes. The further development of tertiary training courses and career pathways for prevention science and its application to policy and practice is important for promoting healthy development in the Asia-Pacific region. This is an important challenge given regional inequalities that demonstrate more severe challenges for tobacco control, improving life expectancy and reducing road trauma in populace areas of the Asia Pacific.

Acknowledgement Sections of this chapter were previously published as: Toumbourou, J.W., Solomon, R., Solomon, S., Soares, A., do Rosario, S., Yong, H., Rowland, B. (in press 2024). The History and Evolution of Health Psychology in the Asia-Pacific region. Chapter 4. In Katherine Brown, Martin Hagger, Cecilia Cheng, Kyra Hamilton and Stephen Sutton (Eds) Sage Handbook of Health Psychology 2nd Edition. And Toumbourou, J.W., Olsson, C., Rowland, B., Renati, S., & Hallam, B. (2014) Health Psychology intervention in key social environments to promote adolescent health. Australian Psychologist. 49, 66–74. https://doi.org/10.1111/ap.12043.

References

Baffsky, R., Ivers, R., Cullen, P., Batterham, P.J., Toumbourou, J.W., Calear, A.L., Werner-Seidler, A., McGillivray, L., Torok, M, (2022) A cluster randomised effectiveness-implementation trial of an intervention to increase the adoption of PAX Good Behaviour Game, a mental health pre-

vention program, in Australian primary schools: Study protocol. Contemporary Clinical Trials Communications. 2022, 100923, https://doi.org/10.1016/j.conctc.2022.100923.
Bartholomew Eldrigde, L. K., Markham, C. M., Ruiter, R. A. C., Fernàndez, M. E., Kok, G., & Parcel, G. S. (2016). Planning health promotion programs: An Intervention Mapping approach (4th ed.). Hoboken, NJ: Wiley.
Berecki-Gisolf, J., Rowland, B., Reavley, N., Minuzzo, B., Toumbourou, J. (2020) Evaluation of community coalition training effects on youth hospital-admitted injury incidence in Victoria, Australia: 2001–2017. Injury Prevention. 26(5), 463-470. https://doi.org/10.1136/injuryprev-2019-043386
Borland R, & Yong H-H. (2018) Tobacco Control: Preventing Smoking and Facilitating Cessation. In: Fisher EB, Cameron LD, Christensen AJ, et al., eds. Principles and Concepts of Behavioral Medicine: A Global Handbook. Springer New York, pp. 771-805.
Browne, J.L., Scibilia, R., Speight, J. (2012) The needs, concerns, and characteristics of younger Australian adults with Type 2 diabetes. Diabetes Medicine. https://doi.org/10.1111/dme.12078.
Catalano, R.F., Fagan, A.A., Gavin, L.E., Greenberg, M.T., Irwin, C.E. Jr., Ross, D.A., Shek, D.T. (2012) Worldwide application of prevention science in adolescent health. Lancet, 379, 1653-1664. https://doi.org/10.1016/S0140-6736(12)60238-4
Catalano, R.F., & Hawkins, J.D. (1996) The social development model: a theory of antisocial behavior. In: J.D. Hawkins, (ed). Delinquency and crime: current theories. New York: Cambridge University Press, pp. 149-197.
Daube, M., & Maddox, R. (2021). Impossible until implemented: New Zealand shows the way. Tobacco Control, 30(4), 361-362. https://doi.org/10.1136/tobaccocontrol-2021-056776
Dessaix A, Maag A, McKenzie J, & Currow DC. (2016) Factors influencing reductions in smoking among Australian adolescents. Public Health Res Pract. 26(1):e2611605. https://doi.org/10.17061/phrp2611605
Doery, E., Satyen, L., Paradies, Y., Rowland, B., Bailey, J.A., Heerde, J.A., Renner, H., Smith, R., & Toumbourou, J. W. (2022) Young adult development indicators for Indigenous and non-Indigenous people: A cross-national longitudinal study. International Journal of Environmental Research and Public Health 19(24), 17084. https://doi.org/10.3390/ijerph192417084
Fulu E, Miedema S, Roselli T, McCook S, Chan KL, Haardörfer R, Jewkes R; UN Multi-country Study on Men and Violence study team. (2017) Pathways between childhood trauma, intimate partner violence, and harsh parenting: findings from the UN Multi-country Study on Men and Violence in Asia and the Pacific. Lancet Global Health. 5(5):e512-e522. https://doi.org/10.1016/S2214-109X(17)30103-1.
Goldfeld S, Bryson H, Mensah F, Gold L, Orsini F, Perlen S, Price A, Hiscock H, Grobler A, Dakin P, Bruce T, Harris D, Kemp L. (2021) Nurse Home Visiting and Maternal Mental Health: 3-Year Follow-Up of a Randomized Trial. Pediatrics. 147(2):e2020025361. https://doi.org/10.1542/peds.2020-025361.
Goldfeld S, Bryson H, Mensah F, Price A, Gold L, Orsini F, Kenny B, Perlen S, Bohingamu Mudiyanselage S, Dakin P, Bruce T, Harris D, Kemp L. (2022) Nurse home visiting to improve child and maternal outcomes: 5-year follow-up of an Australian randomised controlled trial. PLoS One. 17(11):e0277773. https://doi.org/10.1371/journal.pone.0277773.
Green, L., Kreuter, M. (2005) Health program planning: An educational and ecological approach. 4th edition. New York: McGrawhill.
Guerin, N. & White, V. (2020). ASSAD 2017 Statistics & Trends: Australian Secondary Students' Use of Tobacco, Alcohol, Over-the-counter Drugs, and Illicit Substances. Second Edition. Cancer Council Victoria. https://www.health.gov.au/sites/default/files/documents/2020/07/secondary-school-students-use-of-tobacco-alcohol-and-other-drugs-in-2017.pdf
Haggerty, K. P. and McCowan, K. J. (2018) Using the social development strategy to unleash the power of prevention. Journal of the Society for Social Work and Research. 9(4), 741-763. https://www.journals.uchicago.edu/doi/full/10.1086/700274

Hawkins, J.D., Catalano, R.F., Miller, J.Y. (1992) Risk and protective factors for alcohol and other drug problems in adolescence and early adulthood: implications for substance abuse prevention. Psychological Bulletin, 112, 64–105.

Hawkins, J.D., Kosterman, R., Catalano, R.F., Hill, K., Abbot, R.D. (2005) Promoting positive adult functioning through social development intervention in childhood: Long-term effects from the Seattle Social Development Project. Archives of Pediatric and Adolescent Medicine, 159, 25-31. https://doi.org/10.1001/archpedi.162.12.1133

Lang AE, & Braillon A. (2022) Smokefree New Zealand 2025: A Beacon for Global Tobacco and Nicotine Policy Reform. Chest. 162(2):295-296. https://doi.org/10.1016/j.chest.2022.02.021.

Lewis, A., Rowland, B., Tran, A., Solomon, R.F., Patton, G.C., Catalano, R.F., Toumbourou, J.W. (2017) Adolescent Depressive Symptoms in India, Australia and USA: Exploratory Structural Equation Modelling of cross-national invariance and predictions by gender and age. Journal of Affective Disorders. 212, 150–159. https://doi.org/10.1016/j.jad.2017.01.020

Liou L, Joe W, Kumar A, Subramanian SV. (2020) Inequalities in life expectancy: An analysis of 201 countries, 1950-2015. Social Science and Medicine. 253:112964. https://doi.org/10.1016/j.socscimed.2020.112964.

Marshall WE. (2018) Understanding international road safety disparities: Why is Australia so much safer than the United States? Accident Analysis and Prevention. 111: 251-265. https://doi.org/10.1016/j.aap.2017.11.031.

Martin SL, McCann JK, Gascoigne E, Allotey D, Fundira D, Dickin KL. (2020) Mixed-Methods Systematic Review of Behavioral Interventions in Low- and Middle-Income Countries to Increase Family Support for Maternal, Infant, and Young Child Nutrition during the First 1000 Days. Curr Dev Nutr. 4(6):nzaa085. https://doi.org/10.1093/cdn/nzaa085.

Mathers, C. D., & Loncar, D. (2006). Projections of global mortality and burden of disease from 2002 to 2030. *PLOS Medicine*, *3*(11), e442. https://doi.org/10.1371/journal.pmed.0030442

Mathews, L.B., Moodie, M.M., Simmons, A.N., Swinburn, B.A. (2010) The process evaluation of It's Your Move!, an Australian adolescent community-based obesity prevention project. BMC Public Health. https://doi.org/10.1186/1471-2458-10-448.

Meque I, Salom C, Betts KS, Alati R. (2019) Predictors of alcohol use disorders among young adults: A systematic review of longitudinal studies. Alcohol and Alcoholism. 54(3):310-324. https://doi.org/10.1093/alcalc/agz020.

Miller, L., Robertson, N., Allender, S., Nichols, M., Bennett, C., Swinburn, B. (2013) Increasing community capacity and decreasing prevalence of overweight and obesity in a community based intervention among Australian adolescents. Preventive Medicine, 56, 379–384. https://doi.org/2-s2.0-84877588910

Muñoz, R. F., Mrazek, P. J., Haggerty, R. J. (1996) Institute of Medicine report on prevention of mental disorders: Summary and commentary. American Psychologist, 51(11), pp. 1116-1122.

Parks, M., Solomon, R.J., Solomon, S., Rowland, B.C., Hemphill, S.A., Patton, G.C., Toumbourou, J.W. (2020) Delinquency, school context, and risk factors in India, Australia, and the United States: Implications for prevention. Journal of Research on Adolescence. 30(S1), 143-157. https://doi.org/10.1111/jora.12455

Peters SAE, Wang X, Lam TH, Kim HC, Ho S, Ninomiya T, Knuiman M, Vaartjes I, Bots ML, Woodward M; Asia Pacific Cohort Studies Collaboration. (2018) Clustering of risk factors and the risk of incident cardiovascular disease in Asian and Caucasian populations: results from the Asia Pacific Cohort Studies Collaboration. BMJ Open. 8(3):e019335. https://doi.org/10.1136/bmjopen-2017-019335.

Rowland, B., Jonkman, H., Steketee, M., Solomon, R., Solomon, S., Toumbourou, J.W. (2021) A Cross-national comparison of the development of adolescent problem behavior: a 1-year longitudinal study in India, the Netherlands, USA and Australia. Prevention Science. 22, 62–72. https://doi.org/10.1007/s11121-019-01007-3

Rowland, B.C., Kremer, P., Williams, J., Kelly, A.B., Patton, G., Toumbourou, J.W. (2021) A component evaluation of a randomised control community intervention to reduce adolescent alcohol use in Australia. Prevention Science. https://doi.org/10.1007/s11121-021-01310-y

Rowland, B., Kelly, A.B., Mohebbi, M., Kremer, P., Abrahams, C., Abimanyi-Ochom, J., Carter, R., Williams, J., Smith, R., Osborn, A., Hall, J., Hossein, T., Renner, H., Toumbourou, J.W. (2022) Evaluation of Communities That Care - Effects on Municipal Youth Crime Rates in Victoria, Australia: 2010 – 2019. Prevention Science 23(1):24-35. https://doi.org/10.1007/s11121-021-01297-6

Satyen, L., Supol, M., Ranganathan, A., and Toumbourou, J.W. (2020) International and cross-cultural research on men's violence against female intimate partners. Chapter 3 in Todd K. Shackelford (ed.) the SAGE Handbook of Domestic Violence. ISBN: 9781526494863. pp. 40–60. https://uk.sagepub.com/en-gb/eur/the-sage-handbook-of-domestic-violence/book268336#

Schreier, H.M.C., Schonert-Reichl, K.A., Chen, E. (2013) Effect of volunteering on risk factors for cardiovascular disease in adolescents: a randomized controlled trial. JAMA Pediatrics. https://doi.org/10.1007/10.1001/jamapediatrics.2013.1100.

Stubbs T. (2021) Commercial determinants of youth smoking in ASEAN countries: A narrative review of research investigating the influence of tobacco advertising, promotion, and sponsorship. Tobacco Induced Diseases 19:61. https://doi.org/10.1007/10.18332/tid/139124.

Stubbs T, Thomas S, Pitt H, Daube M. (2022) Do health halos and conspicuous consumption influence the appeal and risk perceptions of e-cigarettes among young Cambodian men? Tob Control. 31(4):505-510. https://doi.org/10.1136/tobaccocontrol-2020-056110

Stubbs T, White VM, Kong M, Toumbourou JW. (2022) Uncovering the advertising and promotional strategies of tobacco companies in Cambodia: recall of below-the-line marketing among young male smokers. Tobacco Control. tobaccocontrol-2021-057063. https://doi.org/10.1136/tobaccocontrol-2021-057063.

Stubbs T, White VM, Toumbourou JW. (2022) The influence of cigarette packet branding and colours on young male smokers' recognition, appeal, and harm perceptions of tobacco brands in Cambodia: a mixed-methods study. BMJ Open. 12(9):e064202. https://doi.org/10.1136/bmjopen-2022-064202.

Toumbourou, J.W. (2016) Beneficial action within altruistic and prosocial behavior. Review of General Psychology. 20(3), 245-258. https://doi.org/10.1037/gpr0000081.

Toumbourou, J.W., Hemphill, S.A., Tresidder, J., Humphreys, C., Edwards, J., & Murray, D. (2007). Mental health promotion and socio-economic disadvantage: Lessons from substance abuse, violence and crime prevention and child health. Australian Journal of Health Promotion, 18:3, 184-90. https://doi.org/10.1071/he07184

Toumbourou, J.W., Olsson, C., Rowland, B., Renati, S., & Hallam, B. (2014) Health Psychology intervention in key social environments to promote adolescent health. Australian Psychologist. 49, 66–74. https://doi.org/10.1111/ap.12043

Toumbourou, J.W., Rowland, B., Ghayour-Minaie, M., Sherker, S., Patton, G.C., & Williams, J. (2018). Student survey trends in reported alcohol use and influencing factors in Australia. Drug and Alcohol Review, 37 (S1), S58-S66. https://doi.org/10.1111/dar.12645

Toumbourou, J.W. Rowland, B., Williams, J., Smith, R., & Patton, G.C. (2019) Community intervention to prevent adolescent health behavior problems: Evaluation of Communities that Care in Australia. Health Psychology. 38(6), 536-544. https://doi.org/10.1037/hea0000735

Toumbourou, J. W., White, V., Stubbs, T. (2021). Implementing effective tobacco tax and price policies in low- and middle-income nations: a literature review for Timor Leste. Prepared for the Timor Leste Alliance for Tobacco Control by the Centre for Drug use, Addictive and Anti-social behaviour Research (CEDAAR), Deakin University.

United Nations (2016) Sustainable Development Goals. New York: United Nations.

United Nations (2020) Sustainable Development Goals Progress Report https://unstats.un.org/sdgs/report/2020/goal-03

University of Colorado (2022) Nurse-Family Partnership. Blueprints for Healthy Youth Development. www.blueprintsprograms.org/programs/35999999/nurse-family-partnership/

van de Vijver S, Oti S, Addo J, de Graft-Aikins A, Agyemang C. (2012) Review of community-based interventions for prevention of cardiovascular diseases in low- and middle-income countries. Ethnicity & Health. 651-76. https://doi.org/10.1080/13557858.2012.754409.
Van Ryzin MJ, Fosco GM, Dishion TJ. (2012) Family and peer predictors of substance use from early adolescence to early adulthood: an 11-year prospective analysis. Addict Behav. 37(12):1314-24. doi: https://doi.org/10.1016/j.addbeh.2012.06.020.
Vos, T., Carter, R., Barendregt, J., Mihalopoulos, C., Veerman, J.L., Magnus, A., Cobiac, L., Bertram, M.Y., Wallace, A.L., ACE–Prevention Team (2010) Assessing Cost-Effectiveness in Prevention (ACE–Prevention): Final report. University of Queensland, Brisbane and Deakin University, Melbourne. http://www.sph.uq.edu.au/docs/BODCE/ACE-P/ACE-Prevention_final_report.pdf.
Washington State Institute for Public Policy (2019), Report 716, Other prenatal home visiting programs. Olympia: Washington State Legislature. https://www.wsipp.wa.gov/BenefitCost/Program/716
Wellman RJ, Dugas EN, Dutczak H, O'Loughlin EK, Datta GD, Lauzon B, O'Loughlin J. (2016) Predictors of the Onset of Cigarette Smoking: A Systematic Review of Longitudinal Population-Based Studies in Youth. American Journal of Preventive Medicine. 51(5):767-778. https://doi.org/10.1016/j.amepre.2016.04.003.
Wismans J, Skogsmo I, Nilsson-Ehle A, Lie A, Thynell M, Lindberg G. (2016) Commentary: Status of road safety in Asia. Traffic Injury Prevention.17(3):217-25. https://doi.org/10.1080/15389588.2015.1066498.
World Health Organization (2021). World Health Organization global report on trends in prevalence of tobacco use 2000–2025, fourth edition. Geneva: World Health Organization. https://www.who.int/publications/i/item/9789240039322
World Inequality Lab (2022) World Inequality Report 2022. World Inequality Lab, Paris School of Economics. https://wir2022.wid.world/
Yoong SL, Nathan N, Wolfenden L, Wiggers J, Reilly K, Oldmeadow C, Wyse R, Sutherland R, Delaney T, Butler P, Janssen L, Preece S, Williams CM. (2016) CAFÉ: a multicomponent audit and feedback intervention to improve implementation of healthy food policy in primary school canteens: a randomised controlled trial. International Journal of Behavioral Nutrition and Physical Activity. 13(1):126. https://doi.org/10.1186/s12966-016-0453-z.
Zou X, & Vu HL. (2019) Mapping the knowledge domain of road safety studies: A scientometric analysis. Accident Analysis and Prevention. 132:105243. doi: https://doi.org/10.1016/j.aap.2019.07.019.

John Toumbourou is the Chair in Health Psychology at Deakin University, Australia. He is the Co-Leader of Intervention Science in the Deakin University SEED Lifespan Centre. He has published over 300 peer-refereed papers, which have over 20,000 citations (h-index = 74). He is a prominent researcher and social advocate in areas related to the prevention of alcohol and drug problems and family violence. His research and advocacy led to national reductions in youth alcohol and drug use across Australia and the establishment of the tobacco prevention movement in Timor Leste. In 2023 he received the Presidential Award for lifetime contribution to prevention science research from the Society for Prevention Research.

Bosco Rowland **'s** work history has predominantly focused on designing and evaluating health behaviour interventions and then following participants longitudinally. As a registered psychologist, he has focused primarily on the behaviours of alcohol consumption, smoking, illicit drug use, mental health, and healthy eating. His longitudinal research has focused on how these behaviours change and identifying critical influences on these behaviours at different ages and stages of the life course. He has produced over 100 publications and worked in the not-for-profit, service sector, government, and university settings.

Renati Solomon is an Adjunct Professor in Psychology at Mumbai University, Mumbai, India. His work focuses on psychosocial risk and protective factors, adolescent problem behaviors and positive youth development. He has produced 26 research publications in peer-reviewed journals. As a principal investigator, he has implemented in India, the International Youth Development Study, a longitudinal investigation of the "Communities That Care" youth survey focusing on the behaviors of alcohol consumption, tobacco use, illicit drug use, mental health, and suicide. He has received several national and international awards for his contribution to public health initiatives.

Shree Solomon is a PhD Research Scholar at Martin Luther Christian University, Shillong, India, specializing in Positive Youth Development (PYD). She has co-authored 13 peer-reviewed national and international collaborative papers. Her research focuses on the National Service Scheme (NSS) and its role in achieving the Sustainable Development Goals (SDGs) in India. She has worked as a Project Manager for the International Youth Development Study in India for many years and holds advanced degrees in International Relations and Library and Information Science. She is the recipient of the NIDA International Poster Session Award and the Ford Foundation Doctoral Fellowship.

Afonso Soares is the Director of Policy and Planning within the Timor Leste Ministry of Education. He is a graduate of Deakin University where he completed his Master's degree in Applied Science.

Simao do Rosario is a Project Manager within the United States Aid Organization, Timor Leste. He is an Advisor to the Timor Leste Ministry of Education. He is a graduate of Deakin University where he completed his Master's degree in Applied Science.

Hua-Hie Yong is an Associate Professor of Psychology at Deakin University, Australia. His research focuses on evaluating the impacts of tobacco control policies, understanding the psychosocial determinants of smoking cessation/relapse, and identifying factors influencing the use of nicotine vaping products/e-cigarettes. He has published over 150 peer-reviewed papers (h-index = 55; citations = 10,434). From 2018–2023, he served as the inaugural Policy Research director of the Society for Research on Nicotine and Tobacco online University (SRNT-U), where he contributed to the education of its members.

Bianca Klettke is a Lecturer in the School of Psychology at Deakin University, Australia. She is the inaugural leader of the Cyberpsychology Research Group, and a member of the Intervention Sciences Stream within Deakin's SEED Lifespan Centre. She is a researcher and leading academic in the field of cyberpsychology, particularly technology-facilitated sexual violence. Dr Klettke's recent research has focused on how to keep young people safe online, including online behaviours such as sexting and cyberbullying. Within these areas, Dr Klettke's research has focused on identifying the risk and protective factors of these behaviours. The aim of her research is to help educate various bodies such as governments, schools, community and police services, as well as the parents of children and adolescents in order to promote evidence-based information to inform best outcomes in young people.

Elizabeth Clancy is a Lecturer in Psychology at Deakin University, Australia. Co-lead of the Deakin Cyberpsychology Research Group, and a member of the Intervention Sciences Stream within Deakin's SEED Lifespan Centre. As an early career researcher, her work focus is online behaviours in young adulthood, particularly understanding issues of consent in online relationship behaviours, and the online experiences of trans and gender diverse individuals. She has 46 published papers and has significant experience in collaborations and behavioural interventions.

Adrian Kelly is Associate Professor of Clinical Psychology at Queensland University of Technology, Brisbane, Australia. He is a Fellow of the Clinical College (Australian Psychological

Society), and he also has a Master of Business Administration (University of Queensland). He has published more than 120 papers, many of which have focused on adolescent substance use and linkages to family distress and school connectedness. He has had a significant impact on state government curricula and training relating to adolescent substance use, and he has supervised many postgraduate students in and around evidence-based interventions for substance use.

Jacqueline Allen is a Lecturer working in the School of Criminology and Criminal Justice at Griffith University, Australia. Her research focusses on the development of antisocial behaviour and mental health problems from childhood to young adulthood. These problem domains are often linked through the misuse of drugs and alcohol, studies of which underpin her research agenda. Through her research, Dr Allen strives to understand the normative development of these intertwined problems and to identify opportunities for prevention and intervention.

The Evolution of Drug and Alcohol Consumption Prevention in Colombia

Augusto Pérez-Gómez and Juliana Mejía-Trujillo

Country Context

Colombia is the northernmost country in South America; it has an extension of 1,140,000 km^2, coasts on the Caribbean Sea and the Pacific Ocean, and borders Panama, Venezuela, Brazil, Peru, and Ecuador. It has 52 million inhabitants, three mountain ranges into which the Andes mountain range is separated (western, central, and eastern), by extensive jungles and large plains and has the greatest diversity of birds in the world. The vast majority of the population is of the Catholic religion. Life expectancy at birth is 77 years. Drug trafficking once permeated all civilian life, and even though that situation has changed positively, it is still the main producer of cocaine in the world and Mexico's cartels have been involved in trafficking and export.

Introduction

As in many other Latin American countries, the consumption of illegal psychoactive substances (PAS) in Colombia appears as a phenomenon worthy of mention in the 1960s of the last century, and at that time it was limited almost exclusively to the consumption of marijuana by part of some marginal groups and university students. At that time, the influence of youth movements in the United States exerted an almost magnetic attraction on young people from the rest of the continent—and also on Europeans, of course—and marijuana appeared associated with the famous

A. Pérez-Gómez (✉) · J. Mejía-Trujillo
Corporación Nuevos Rumbos, Bogotá, Colombia
e-mail: aperez@nuevosrumbos.org; jmejia@nuevosrumbos.org

A. Pérez-Gómez, J. Mejía-Trujillo (eds.), *Drug Abuse Prevention*, Advances in Mental Health and Addiction, https://doi.org/10.1007/978-3-031-99621-4_3

gesture of "peace and love." At the same time, it is discovered that two Colombian varieties, the so-called Golden Santa Marta and Punto Rojo have an excellent quality that is highly sought after by North Americans: then begins what would become the first wave of drug trafficking.

After several years of drawing attention to the increase in cases related to substance use, in 1985 Colombia had its first national plan for the prevention of drug use, in which several ministries and the Colombian Institute of Family Welfare participated, with the support of the United Nations Office on Drugs and Crime, known at that time as UNFDAC (currently UNODC). In fact, that was the only national plan on drug consumption that has existed in the country: different governments have indicated that the problem is of national interest from the point of view of public health, but in reality only one government (that of Andrés Pastrana, 1998–2002) gave priority to the issue, creating a presidential council with the name of Rumbos, which made it possible to develop public policies, propose a law on prevention as a matter of state and not of governments, and create nearly 220 municipal committees responsible for leading prevention actions with clear guidelines. Unfortunately, the following government dismantled what had been achieved due to lack of interest. That is the story that is repeated over and over again throughout our continent.

Evolution of Public Policies

Historical Background at the Legislative Level

Even though the indigenous populations of Colombia have always used substances that modify states of consciousness and mood (yajé, mambeo of coca leaves, fermented drinks), in general it can be said that such practices have never represented a problem to the extent that they are associated with the rites of those cultures. On the contrary, the abusive consumption of alcohol has a long history, of which there are illustrative documents since the seventeenth century, when the president of the Royal Court of Santa Fé de Bogotá, Dionisio Pérez Manrique de Lara tried without success to prohibit the production, sale, and consumption of chicha.[1] A century later, in 1748, the Church and the state joined forces to issue a royal decree with the same objective, and with the same results. Simón Bolívar himself, in 1820, issued a decree threatening those who sold chicha with expropriation of property and expatriation. The results were equally poor (Bejarano, 1950).

A tight summary of the most important regulations of the last century would include the following (Table 1):

[1] In Colombia, chicha is a drink derived from the fermentation of corn, but the same name is used in other countries on the continent to refer to fermented fruit or cereal drinks, and even non-alcoholic drinks.

Table 1 Regulations in Colombia

Type of regulations	Id	Year	Object
Law	11	1920	It restricted the formulation of medicines to doctors and pharmacists
Law	118	1928	It included the term "misuse" of drugs but did not impose penalties on offenders
Penal Code Article	210	1936 (until 1980)	Sanctioned the production, distribution, and trafficking of narcotics; It did not include marijuana or cocaine, nor did it sanction their use
Ministerial Resolution	25	1938 (February 11)	It restricted the sale of coca leaves to authorized pharmacies and drugstores and only under medical prescription
Resolution	578	1941	He ordered a census of coca plantations and prohibited the planting of new crops
Law	45	1946	It penalized the cultivation and conservation of coca plants
Decree	846	1947	It was the first statute against coca and marijuana: it prohibited paying wages in coca leaves, cultivating, distributing, and selling both plants, imposed criminal sanctions on those who possessed morphine, heroin, and other narcotics and imposed fines and prison sentences on those who violate these provisions. This law was never applied
Law	3.4	1948	It regulated the consumption and production of chicha
Decree	14	1955	It reaffirmed the mixed system of sanctions of the Penal Code of 1936
Law	30	1986 (currently)	The National Narcotics Council was created. It focused fundamentally on matters related to supply control and of 97 articles, only a few were dedicated to matters related to demand (prevention in the educational environment, sanctions, mandatory treatment—the latter was modified by a constitutional ruling)
Ruling of the Constitutional Court	C221	1994	It was stated that no one could be punished for using, and no adult could be forced to undergo treatment for that reason
Decree	1108	1994	Regulates ruling C221: prohibition of consumption in public places by pregnant women and minors
Decree	2193	1998	It advocated the design of policies that would contribute to creating the conditions for the prevention and reduction of the consumption of psychoactive substances
Ministry of Health Resolution	2358	1998	It was the first sectoral policy that specified the obligation to prevent the misuse of psychoactive substances
Decree	1943	1999	It modified the structure of the National Narcotics Directorate and the Presidential Program for Coping with the Consumption of Psychoactive Substances

(continued)

Table 1 (continued)

Type of regulations	Id	Year	Object
Ministry of Health Resolution	1315	2006	The standards for the authorization of treatment centers were defined.
Law	1098	2006	Children are protected from the consumption of SPA and its use in the manufacturing and marketing process of SPA is prohibited
Law	1109	2006	Protected from the effects of tobacco through the approval of the WHO framework agreement for Colombia
Law	1335	2009	Anti-tobacco law. Policies were formulated to prevent, avoid, and abandon tobacco consumption
Legislative act	002	2009	Prohibits the carrying and consumption of SPA, modifying article 49 of the constitution
Decree	120	2010	Minors who consume must attend a course on the prevention of SPA consumption
Decree	2897	2011	Creation of the coordination of the "fight against illicit drugs" policy, through the creation of the Anti-Drug Policy Directorate
Law	1438	2011	The General Health Social Security System is reformed and makes promotion and prevention the main axis of public health actions
Ruling of the Constitutional Court	C574	2011	It declares unconstitutional the Legislative Act 002/2009, which prohibited the possession and consumption of drugs
Law	1566	2012	Turns the problem of SPA consumption into a public health issue
Resolution	1441	2013	It completely medicalized the drug problem and produced a national reaction of rejection
Resolution	2003	2014	Corrected the errors of resolution 1441 of 2013
Resolution	429	2016	The Comprehensive Health Care Policy is promulgated
Resolution	3202	2016	The comprehensive care path for substance use disorders is built
Law	1801 (art. 34)	2016	National Police and Coexistence Code. In his article he established sanctions for consuming substances in public spaces
Decree	1844	2018	It regulates the Police Code. Provides for the destruction of the carried substances
Resolution	4886	2018	A new mental health policy is adopted, with emphasis on early intervention
Law	2000	2019	It specifies the sanctions of the Police Code for consumption in educational spaces, surrounding areas, and in public spaces. Drug Addiction Care Centers (CAD) are created
Resolution	2404	2019	Established the need to carry out a psychosocial risk assessment, including substance use

(continued)

Table 1 (continued)

Type of regulations	Id	Year	Object
Ministry of Health Resolution	89	2019	Formulates the comprehensive policy for the prevention and care of SPA consumption
Resolution of the National Narcotics Council	003	2022	Gives mayors power to define consumption spaces for adults
Presidential decree	2114	2023	Repeals police code rule that prohibited possession and sale of drugs
Law	325	2024	Cigarettes and vapes are regulated at the same level as traditional cigarettes

Diagnostic

There Is a Lack of Financing for the Implementation of Public Policies on Demand Control and the Execution of Preventive Programs

Even though some important political guidelines were presented in 2009 (National Drug Demand Reduction Commission, 2008), the reality is that the impact of these policies was minimal because neither at the central nor at the municipal level were resources allocated to turn it into concrete actions. The impression that emerges consistently from the actions of successive governments is that drug use is not considered an issue that should be given any degree of priority, despite the fact that it is recognized that it affects a large number of people (about 500,000 would need treatment, according to the latest national study, especially minors). Regarding investments, 98% of the resources go to supply control, and less than 2% to demand reduction. We have been implementing it for 10 years, with state financing, the Familias Fuertes preventive program, but with very low coverage due to its very high costs, the conditions of access to the program, and its excessive duration. The choice of this program does not seem to have been a very fortunate decision.

There Is a Great Delay in Addressing the Problem of Drug Consumption

One of the great difficulties in Colombia is the lack of consistency in the execution of prevention and treatment strategies. Although a large number of initiatives have been taken to develop preventive programs, especially at the private level, very few of them have been evaluated with any rigor, and their dissemination is minimal. According to Corrêa et al. (2021), in more than 400 publications on Colombian preventive programs, only four refer to evaluations. And in the field of treatment the situation is no better: treatment strategies and centers have not been evaluated in the country for many years, with very few exceptions.

The Allocation of Resources to Evaluate the Dimensions of the Problem

In most countries in the hemisphere, national studies are carried out with the population aged 12 to 65 every four years, and in the interim, studies are carried out with the school-going population. In Colombia, a study was carried out in 1996 (Ministry of Justice &National Directorate of Narcotics, 1996), the next in 2008 (Ministry of Social Protection, CICAD & National Directorate of Narcotics, 2009), then in 2013 (Ministry of Justice and Law & Ministry of Health and Social Protection, 2014), and in 2019. This last study has serious methodological errors, and its results are counter-evident: there would have been a decrease in consumption without any intervention. The studies with the school population were carried out in 2004, 2011, 2016 (published in 2018), and 2022 (Ministry of Social Protection & CICAD, 2004; Ministries of Education, Justice and Law, Health and Social Protection & CICAD, 2012, 2018 and 2023).

Apart from these studies, the Nuevos Rumbos Corporation carried out three studies on alcohol consumption in minors (see Pérez-Gómez & Scoppetta, 2009; Pérez-Gómez et al., 2015, 2021). All three can be consulted at www.nuevosrumbos.org.

There Is no Stability in the Structures of the State That Guarantees Continuity in Actions

The state structures we refer to include four components: norms and laws; the institutions; the qualification of the people involved; and allocated resources. We have already seen what the situation of the regulations is, full of disparate elements and lacking a common thread in many cases, or inapplicable due to the enormous amount of resources that their implementation requires. Regarding institutions, the core of attention to the problem of drug consumption is located in the Ministry of Health and Social Protection with regard to treatment, and in the Ministry of Justice with regard to prevention. Regarding professional qualification in the responsible institutions, all too often there is a lack of qualified personnel to assume these functions. And, finally, the resources allocated at the central level are neither relevant nor sufficient to respond to the most basic demands of the population.

However, it must be said that starting in 2016 the social security system assumed the costs of care at the level of treatment for consumption, especially using the network of private entities, since government entities are usually intended to provide care emergencies; an exception is Carisma, in Medellín, which is one of the most advanced centers in the country. At the outpatient level, the system offers the possibility of having up to 10 individual sessions, but it is not guaranteed that the appointments will be with the same professional: so, even though there is progress, there is still much to be specified.

The government that began in August 2022 proposed a radical change to the entire drug policy in the country, including everything related to health. Yes, some changes have been made, but there is great skepticism among the population, which interprets that many benefits are being given to people who in any other country would be considered simply dangerous criminals. The changes in the field of health are not clear, and the reform proposal faces very marked opposition. The only thing that stands out is the importance that would be given to harm reduction.

Prevention Activities

Preventive Actions

In 1984, the government began structuring the National Drug Addiction Prevention Plan (PNPD), with the support of the United Nations office equivalent to the current UNODC, which at that time was called UNFDAC (United Nations Fund for Drug Abuse Control), which was approved in 1985. In this plan, under the coordination of the Presidency of the Republic, in addition to National Planning and the National Council on Narcotic Drugs, the Colombian Institute of Family Welfare (ICBF), and the Ministries of Education, Health, Justice, Agriculture, and Communications. This plan, which lasted with ups and downs until the beginning of 1994, sought especially inter-institutional coordination, an objective that unfortunately was not achieved except in a very superficial way.

Despite this, Colombia became the leader in the region and contributed substantially to the creation of CICAD (Inter-American Commission for Drug Abuse Control) by the Organization of American States (OAS) in 1986.

In this plan, it was the Ministry of Education that developed the greatest number of activities and also proposed a profound transformation in the educational community, which in reality did not occur. However, the approach to drug consumption prevention soon became "prevention of socially relevant problems," understanding that the basis of drug consumption was common to other problems such as juvenile delinquency, teenage pregnancy, and school dropout. These reflections would be widely validated by systematic research in numerous countries, and are currently still considered correct, under the name of "behavioral predictors approach," which includes the identification of risk and protective factors.

The work of the Ministry of Education resulted in the adoption of the concept of "comprehensive prevention," which suggested a holistic approach to the drug problem: it proposed to analyze in an articulated manner what was related to illicit crops, the sale of inputs, drug trafficking, money laundering, prevention of consumption, treatment, and rehabilitation. However, reality has shown that issues related to what has been misleadingly called the "supply" and "demand" of drugs require completely different approaches (National Advisory Commission on Drug Policy, 2015).

The actions carried out were never subject to systematic evaluations, and most of what remains are oral and photographic records, but there are few published documents. However, it is indisputable that what happened between 1985 and 1990 left traces that have not yet been erased, as they marked the path that would lead, little by little, to CICAD unifying work criteria for the entire region, both in the field of prevention as well as research.

Apart from CICAD's initiative to unify work criteria for the entire region, there was no unity of concepts or strategies at government levels. In fact, most of the prevention actions in Colombia have been developed, in these 35 years, by non-governmental entities. Some of the main examples are the La Casa Program of the Universidad de los Andes in Bogotá; Roads, in Cali; Arise in Medellín; and the Universidad del Norte in Barranquilla. All of these institutions tried to work with the educational community and some with the community in general. But upon losing the support of government entities, and in some cases international entities, their actions began to disappear.

Rumbos (1998–2002), the presidential program to which we alluded at the beginning of this chapter, made it possible to place drug consumption as one of the 10 priority problems of the country. During those four years, the Municipal Committees on Psychoactive Substances were constantly stimulated and supported, international help was sought to support specific prevention projects, 16 research projects were developed, the largest study of drug use among young people on the continent was carried out (more than 200,000 people participated) and effective coordination was carried out between different government agencies (RUMBOS, 2002).

Between 2002 and 2010, no preventive activities were carried out with national leadership, and some specific and local actions of very low impact were simply developed. From 2011 to the present, government investments continue to be very marginal, even though, especially at the level of municipalities and cities; there is concern about the increase in consumption and other associated problems, such as school dropouts, the connection of young people to criminal gangs, teenage pregnancy, among others.

Preventive Programs

In 2012, the Nuevos Rumbos Corporation carried out an inventory of the preventive programs used in Colombia, and that had some type of evaluation, in order to make them available to the communities and thus implement those that had the best results. In that search, 14 programs were found, of which only some are still being implemented; In fact, it is striking that in 2024 there are fewer programs available than back then.

Social Competence and School Health

It is a program that has been developed since 2000 as part of the practical training of undergraduate students, and is aimed at the development of a spiral curriculum (from preschool to 11th, with weekly sessions) through which schoolchildren are encouraged to the development of socio-emotional skills according to each moment of life, so that they have the necessary elements to take care of their mental health, reject, and delay the start of consumption, and develop support networks. It has three versions: Coexistence, for children transitioning to 3rd grade, to address basic skills; Typical, for children of 4th to 7th grade, where life skills are taught; and Arcos, 8th to 11th grade, where transition skills are worked on (Flórez-Alarcón and Vélez-Botero, 2020).

CEMA-PEMA Also created by the Lifestyle and Human Development Research Group of the National University of Colombia in 2001, it is a group intervention that seeks to reduce alcohol consumption in adolescents and young people between 12 and 25 years old in the school environment and university. It has six sessions and is considered selective prevention. It is supported by brief motivational intervention, skills training, and self-control in order to promote self-determination to avoid consumption or the adoption of self-care and mutual care guidelines (Ramírez et al., 2014).

ConSentidos/SanaMente It is a selective preventive program that directly addresses the issue of alcohol and cigarettes (and marijuana in the fifth level of the program), and at the same time promotes the development of basic skills for coping with peer pressure, the conceptualization of friendship as a protective relationship, the breadth of the perception of values, the strengthening of critical analysis of media messages, the promotion and strengthening of family skills that increase their capacity for containment and assertiveness against consumption. It is a program that is inserted into the school curriculum, developed by the Collective Here and Now since 2006, and aimed at students from 5th to 9th grade, the parents of these children, and adolescents and their teachers. (Colectivo Aquí y Ahora, 2012).

SanaMente is a version of ConSentidos but aimed at students between 9 and 11 years old belonging to schools from low socioeconomic strata (Colectivo Aquí y Ahora, 2012).

Anímate Created by the Buscando Ánimo Corporation in 1999, it is a program that is developed in the school environment and is aimed at students from 6th to 11th grade. It seeks to create conditions to strengthen protective factors against the risk of suicide and SPA consumption. The in-class workshops, guided by the course director, have three components: group work, plenary discussion, and individual work. It is the only program that carried out periodic evaluation for more than 15 years, with positive results in reducing lifetime, year and month prevalence of drug use (Aja Eslava & Gómez Avila, 2013).

Retomemos It is a program of the Surgir Corporation and is based on the development of life skills and the promotion of the acquisition of healthy lifestyles, as a protective strategy against vulnerability to the consumption of licit and illicit psychoactive substances in young people. It is aimed at students, teachers, and parents (Sugir Corporation, 2011).

Familias Fuertes It is an adaptation of the American program Strengthening Families. The goal of FF is to reduce the prevalence of adolescent risk behaviors by strengthening family ties.

With adults, the goal is the acquisition of emotional connection skills, promoting support and proximity to their children, as well as effective ways to discipline, guide, and inform; treat effectively; and listen to their children with empathy. In adolescents, the aim is to achieve better communication with their parents, make healthy decisions, and avoid risky behaviors; develop effective skills to avoid risky behaviors, cope with stress and peer pressure, choose good friends, and display prosocial behavior; and develop life projects.

The program consists of seven intervention sessions with families to build protection strategies for both adolescents and their parents. Ideally, each teenager attends with two adults, either his/her parents or one of them, and another adult who is part of the teenager's life (uncle, grandfather, good friend of the family). The program includes a series of resources: teaching manuals, models for individual and group practices, as well as role-playing games, role reversals, and videos to illustrate the topics.

It is based on ecological models, behavior change, effective parenting, goal setting theory, and community organization models.

Despite being an expensive program that is based on working with solid families, it is the only program that has been formally adopted by the Colombian state.

IBEM The preventive program based on Brief Intervention and Motivational Interviewing (IBEM), developed by Corporación Nuevos Rumbos since 2012 to work with adolescents, allows identifying a problem with alcohol consumption or other SPA, whether present or latent, mobilizing the individual towards change through increased motivation; likewise, it seeks to promote and reinforce non-consumption in those who are not interested or who for various reasons have never consumed. Its application includes all students in grades 8 and 9. It is worth mentioning that each of these meetings is individual and lasts approximately 15 min.

The preventive intervention is made up of three meetings, separated by three months between each one: the first is detection and interview about the situation that the young person is experiencing; motivation is investigated, support is provided in the search for goal(s) and strategies that allow you to modify frequency, quantity, or consumption habits; and a session closure is carried out announcing the next meeting in three months. In the second, monitoring is carried out to analyze achievements and difficulties; and in the third, a new follow-up is carried out and the process is closed.

Although IBEM has shown to have positive effects through efficacy and effectiveness evaluations with the school population (Reyes-Rodríguez et al., 2018, 2020), efforts have been made to continue its adaptation to the university population of various regions and characteristics. The IBEM-U preventive program (Brief Intervention based on Motivational Interviewing in its modality for university students) is aimed at preventing the abusive consumption of alcohol in undergraduate or graduate students. IBEM-U allows you to identify a problem with the consumption of this substance, using validated instruments, and from there determine one of four risk levels (Low, Medium, High, or Severe) for each participant. Each one is motivated to set a goal and strategies that allow them to reduce the amount and frequency of use, as well as promote low-risk alcohol consumption, and even abstinence, if they wish.

Comunidades Que se Cuidan (CQC)

The Comunidades Que se Cuidan® (CQC) system is a name registered by the Corporación Nuevos Rumbos, to refer to the Colombian version of Communities That Care (CTC), created by the University of Washington more than 30 years ago, and which has undergone numerous adjustments and updates. CQC provides an operational framework to help the community build positive, healthy futures for its young people, through a community action model that is based on years of research and continuous improvement. The system is based on the public health approach and the social development model, and seeks to prevent five problems in children and adolescents: the consumption of alcohol and other psychoactive substances, delinquency, teenage pregnancy, school dropouts, and violence.

Caring Communities is implemented in more than 11 countries around the world. In Latin America, Nuevos Rumbos is the only entity that has developed the preventive system in Colombia and Chile (Mejía-Trujillo & Pérez-Gómez, 2023). In Brazil, measures are being taken to implement it from 2024.

The Comunidades Que se Cuidan (CQC) is considered a preventive system and not a program, because its definition, foundation, and structuring are based on the scientific postulates developed in recent decades by prevention science. This system allows the development, through a well-defined methodology, of community articulation processes that, based on real data on the community profile, contribute to the identification of risk and protection factors associated with problems specific to young people and adolescents (Hawkins & Catalan).

CQC has five phases:

1. Beginning: the readiness for change in the community is evaluated, actors are identified, leaders are recruited, and support is obtained from schools to apply the survey on protective and risk factors.
2. Organize, introduce, engage: a coalition is formed and key adult actors are trained; a vision of the future is developed for the children of the community and a structure is organized to be able to move in that direction. Two training sessions are provided: guidance for leaders on prevention and how to organize a Community Board that is the highest authority when making decisions.
3. Development of a community profile: a phase in which the survey is applied to young people. The chosen leaders receive training on how to interpret protective and risk factors and on that basis suggest which ones are priorities. Existing

community programs, policies, and resources addressing protective and risk factors are also evaluated.
4. Community planning: the Community Board reviews the results of Phase 3 and develops an action plan, based on training in community planning. Programs are chosen that can change risk factors and problem behaviors. Measurable goals and objectives are proposed.
5. Implementation, evaluation, and monitoring: training is offered for the execution of the community plan considering the importance of remaining faithful to the guidelines of the system, the financial aspects of implementation, and the elements that will allow the results to be adequately evaluated.

Encaminándolos hacia Buenas Decisiones (EBD)

In English *Guiding Good Choices* is a preventive program from the University of Washington in Seattle (United States) (Scheuer et al., 2022), which in Colombia is implemented by the Nuevos Rumbos Corporation. It is developed in order to train parents of children between the ages of 9 and 14 in family skills and its central objective is to teach parents how to reduce the risk of their children presenting difficulties with the consumption of psychoactive substances and delinquent behavior.

"Guiding Good Choices" focuses on strengthening protective factors in the family to reduce the presence of problematic behaviors, in addition to generating support networks among participating families, and to support their parenting and family development processes.

The program has five sessions, lasting approximately 2 hours per week, which are suggested to be done every 8–15 days. The total number of families per session can range between 10 and 15 families maximum.

Publications and Research

In Colombia, research on drug consumption and treatment has never been abundant. When looking at the set of publications, most of them have to do with prevalence of consumption, and range from national studies that began in the 1990s of the last century, to numerous micro studies carried out in small populations or in isolated educational institutions. The latter do not provide any overview of the national scenario: they only show that alcohol is the most consumed substance, followed by tobacco and marijuana.

In this section we will review the studies grouping them into four categories: studies on consumption (prevalence), studies evaluating prevention programs and strategies, evaluations of treatments, and others. The latter includes projects such as transitions in drug use, female identity and drugs, association between drug use and physical illnesses, use of electronic cigarettes and vaping devices, and impact of alcohol and other substance consumption on families' quality of life (Tables 2, 3, and 4).

Conclusions and Recommendations

The problem of drug consumption in Colombia has never followed a coherent line. Although different governments have undertaken activities aimed at stopping the growth of consumption, in the vast majority of cases it has been about weak measures, poorly thought out and poorly executed advertising campaigns, programs with low coverage and lacking evaluation, or the selection of a program whose excessive costs limit its effectiveness or its application. In mid-2024 the situation is very confusing: despite two years of new government, not a single decision has been made nor investments made in this field. The new policy, weak and poorly formulated, talks about working with homeless people and juvenile delinquents, doing harm reduction and mitigation. In this way, only a few thousand cases would be covered, but it would ignore that prevention is the fundamental pillar of all public health policy. We can only hope that the mayors of the main cities assume the responsibility of facing a reality that cannot be hidden: consumption increases, extends to rural areas, and ends up becoming a problem of citizen security, as it is well known that drugs, alcohol abuse, crime, and violence feed each other, in an endless vicious circle. In Colombia, the vast majority of prevention activities are undertaken by private organizations, with unquestionable good intentions but often without adequate training. As we show in the chapter, there are currently fewer preventive programs in the country than there were 10 years ago, and although awareness of the importance of having properly evaluated programs has increased, there are no internally available resources to do so.

It is necessary to create a governing body that, based on state policies (not governments, as has always happened), organizes actions, stimulates research, favors the adequate training of those who will assume the actions, promotes the communities jointly with state entities, and assumes responsibility for managing the problem.

Table 2 Studies on psychoactive substances in Colombia

Issue	Year	Authors	Conclusions
Self-reported consumption of illegal psychoactive substances in a street population in Cali-Colombia	2015	Hernández-Carrillo et al.	Study carried out in 2010; a high level of marijuana and basuco consumption is shown
Prevalence and variables associated with the consumption of psychoactive substances in Colombian men self-identified as homosexuals	2015	Pineda	It shows a high alcohol consumption and a greater probability of consumption of other SPA in this population
Second study on alcohol consumption in children under 18 years of age in seven departmental capitals and two small cities	2015	Pérez-Gómez et al.	It shows that underage drinking has decreased since 2009, but is still very high
III Andean epidemiological study on drug consumption in the university population of Colombia	2016	UNODC and Minjusticia	Shows the magnitude of SPA consumption in university students
Study of psychoactive substance consumption in the Adolescent Criminal Responsibility System (ACRS)	2017	Ministry of Justice et al.	Adolescents within the System of Criminal Responsibility have a much higher consumption of SPA, especially illicit ones, than the school population
Prevalence and factors associated with alcohol consumption in young people from poor homes in the Montes de María subregion, in the Colombian Caribbean	2018	Salcedo-Mejía et al.	A very high alcohol consumption is found in this population
Substance use in adolescents and its association with risk and protective factors in Colombia	2018	Montero Zamora et al.	The validity of the risk and protective factors within the CQC preventive system is demonstrated
National Study of Psychoactive Substance Consumption in school population in Colombia, 2016	2018	MinJusticia et al.	It shows an increase in the consumption of different substances among adolescents
Profiles associated with alcohol consumption in Colombian adolescents	2018	Pérez-Gómez et al.	The differences between adolescents who have high and low alcohol consumption are shown
National Study on the Consumption of Psychoactive Substances Colombia, 2019	2019	Minjusticia and DANE	The data from this study would indicate a significant decrease in drug consumption in Colombia. It has serious methodological errors
Consumption of alcohol, tobacco, and psychoactive substances by adolescents in an indigenous territory in the Colombian Amazon	2020	Pedroza-Buitrago et al.	This population has a higher consumption of SPA, with the exception of cocaine and inhalants, than the national average
Study of psychoactive substance consumption in Bogotá, DC	2022	Mayor's Office of Bogotá	Updates information on SPA consumption in the capital district

(continued)

Table 2 (continued)

Issue	Year	Authors	Conclusions
Third study on alcohol consumption in children under 18 years of age in Colombia	2022	Pérez-Gómez et al.	Shows the evolution of alcohol consumption during the Covid-19 pandemic
National Study on the Consumption of Psychoactive Substances in the school population in Colombia, 2022	2022	MinJustica and MinEducación	Shows the evolution of consumption in high school students
Consumption of psychoactive substances in the young population during the context of preventive social isolation in Medellín, Colombia, 2020	2023	Gomez et al.	A decrease in consumption prevalence is evident during the Covid-19 pandemic

Table 3 Studies on prevention programs and strategies in Colombia

Issue	Year	Authors	Conclusions
Implementation and adaptation in Colombia of the Communities That Care preventive system	2015	Mejía-Trujillo et al.	The differences between CTC and CQC, the cut-off points and the adaptation process in Colombia are shown
Evaluation of a program for the prevention of psychoactive substance use for children	2015	Hernandez	Mediating factors in substance use were identified through an evaluation with parents, students, and teachers
Effectiveness of a Brief Intervention based on Motivational Interviews in Colombian adolescents (IBEM)	2018	Reyes-Rodriguez et al.	IBEM reduces the frequency and quantity of alcohol consumption in high school students
The evaluation of a program (Sanamente) in Colombia to prevent alcohol consumption. Lessons learned	2019	Martínez et al.	It influences the perception of risk and the normative influences perceived by adolescents
Evaluation of the prevention program "Brief Intervention based on Motivational Interviews" in Colombian adolescents	2020	Reyes-Rodriguez et al.	The effects of the intervention occur mainly between the first and second encounters and are maintained until the third
Evaluation of the prevention program: "Strong Families: Love and limits" in Colombia	2020	Castaño-Perez	Changes were observed in parental behavior, but not in adolescent risk behaviors
Effectiveness of a program for the prevention of psychoactive substance consumption in university students	2023	Cogollo-Milanés et al.	The program was effective in reducing alcohol consumption and curbing marijuana and cocaine use
Ten years of implementation of the Communities That Care for themselves preventive system in Colombia	2023	Mejía-Trujillo & Pérez-Gómez	CQC is shown to be a viable program for Latin America

Table 4 Other studies in Colombia

Issue	Year	Authors	Conclusions
Consumption of psychoactive substances and violent behaviors in students from 11 to 18 years old in Itagüí, Colombia	2015	Chavarriaga-Ríos & Segura-Cardona	There is an association between violent behavior and SPA use
Mental disorders and drug consumption in the population victims of the armed conflict in three cities in Colombia	2017	Castaño et al.	Mental disorders and SPA consumption in this population are higher than in the general population
Factors associated with the consumption of substances of abuse in pregnant patients	2018	Mejia et al.	An association was found between consumption during pregnancy with abandonment of the couple, violence, and a history of psychiatric illness
Mental health and psychoactive substance use in Colombian adolescents	2018	Cruz-Ramirez et al.	The adolescent population with affect disorders has higher risks of consuming SPA
Stages of behavioral change regarding the consumption of psychoactive substances in schoolchildren from 9 to 17 years of age in Bogotá, DC, Colombia	2019	Núñez et al.	Examines the stages of Proshaska and DiClementi's transtheoretical model in a group of Bogotá students
Adaptation of the Questionnaire for Identification of Disorders Due to Alcohol Consumption (AUDIT) in Colombian university students	2019	Riveros et al.	The study shows that the AUDIT has adequate psychometric conditions
Association between psychoactive substance abuse and health disorders in Colombian problem drug users: second study	2020	Pérez-Gómez et al.	The association between drug consumption and neurological, gastric, cognitive, and pulmonary damage is shown
Feasibility of implementing alcohol health literacy tests in Colombia	2021	Scoppetta et al.	The greater the risk due to alcohol consumption, the greater the openness to discussing the issue with health professionals
Costs of an alcohol measurement intervention in three Latin American countries	2022	Solovei et al.	The costs of implementing a screening program in primary health care are lower in Colombia than in Mexico or Peru
Country and policy factors influencing the implementation of primary care-based alcohol screening: a comparison of Colombia, Mexico, and Peru	2023	Kokole et al.	Considering alcohol consumption as a public health issue contributes to increasing the number of screenings
How much does it cost the family for one of its members to be a drug and alcohol user	2023	Pérez-Gómez et al.	Having a drug user in the family affects expenses up to 6 times the monthly budget, and up to 13 times if indirect costs are included

References

Aja Eslava, L., & Gómez Avila, J. (2013). Evaluación y seguimiento de un programa de prevención de consumo de SPA y riesgo de suicidio: 1999—2012. *Tipica Boletín electrónico de Salud Escolar*, *9*(2).

Alcaldía Mayor de Bogotá, Secretaría Distrital de Salud de Bogotá & Oficina de las Naciones Unidas contra la Droga y el Delito (2022). Estudio de consumo de sustancias psicoactivas en Bogotá D.C., 2022.

Bejarano, J. (1950). *La derrota de un vicio: Origen e historia de la chicha*. Iqueima.

Castaño, G. A., Sierra, G., Sánchez, D. A. M., Torres, Y., Salas, C., & Buitrago, C. (2017). Trastornos mentales y consumo de drogas en la población víctima del conflicto armado en tres ciudades de Colombia. *Biomedica*, *38*, 77-92. doi:https://doi.org/10.7705/biomedica.v38i0.3890

Castaño-Pérez, G., Salas, C., & Buitrago, C. (2020). Evaluation of the prevention program: "strong families: Love and limits" in Colombia. International Journal of Mental Health and Addiction, 18(2), 459-470

Chavarriaga-Ríos, M. C., & Segura-Cardona, Á. (2015). Consumo de sustancias psicoactivas y comportamientos violentos en estudiantes de 11 a 18 años. Itagüí, Colombia. *Revista de salud publica*, *17*(5), 655-666. https://doi.org/10.15446/rsap.v17n5.31366

Cogollo-Milanés, Z., Gómez-Bustamante, E. & Campo-Arias, A. (2023). Efectividad de un programa para la prevención de consumo de sustancias psicoactivas en estudiantes universitarios. Revista Facultad Nacional de Salud Pública, 41 (3), e04. https://doi.org/10.17533/udea.rfnsp.e351578

Colectivo Aquí y Ahora. (2012). *Consentidos—Programa de prevención selectivo del consumo de alcohol, cigarrillo y otras drogas*. http://www.consentidos.org/

Comisión Nacional de Reducción de la Demanda de Drogas. (2008). *Política Integral para la Prevención y Atención del Consumo de Sustancias Psicoactivas*. Gobierno de Colombia.

Comisión Nacional Asesora en Política de Drogas. (2015). Informe Final. Bogotá.

Corrêa, A., Wells, A., Guidi Gentil, C., & Brown, E. C. (2021) Results of a *Systematic Review of Preventive Interventions for Youth Alcohol, Tobacco and Other Drug Use in Latin American and the Caribbean*. Report to the Organization of American States, Inter-American Drug Abuse Control Commission. University of Miami.

Corporación Sugir. (2011). *Retomemos: Una propuesta para tomar en serio*. http://www.corporacionsurgir.org/surgir/index.php/programas-y-proyectos/retomemos

Cruz-Ramírez, V., Gómez-Restrepo, C., & Rincón, C. J. (2018). Salud Mental Y Consumo De Sustancias Psicoactivas En Adolescentes Colombianos. Health & Addictions/Salud y Drogas, 18(1).

Flórez-Alarcón y Vélez-Botero. (2020). Competencia social y salud escolar OJO TERMINAR

Gómez Velásquez, S., M.A. Quirós Vélez, J.A. Matta Herrera, D.A. Ossa Estrada, y M. Giraldo Torres (2023). Consumo de sustancias psicoactivas en población joven durante el contexto de aislamiento social preventivo en Medellín, Colombia 2020. Revista de la Universidad de La Salle, (90), 249-272.

Hawkins, D., & Catalano, R. (2002). OJO COMPLETAR

Hernández-Carrillo, M., Álvarez-Claros, K. E., & Osorio-Sabogal, I. A. (2015). Consumo autoreportado de sustancias psicoactivas ilegales en una población habitante de calle de Cali-Colombia. Revista de Salud Pública, 17(2), 217-228. https://doi.org/10.15446/rsap.v17n2.30016

Hernández-Ramírez, EM, (2015). Evaluación de un programa de prevención del consumo de sustancias psicoactivas para la infancia. Salud y drogas, 15 (1), 67-77.

Kokole, D., Mercken, L., Anderson, P., Mejía-Trujillo, J., Pérez-Gómez, A. et al., (2023). Country and policy factors influencing the implementation of primary care-based alcohol screening: a comparison of Colombia, Mexico and Peru. Global Public Health 18(1) 2207410 doi:https://doi.org/10.1080/17441692.2023.2207410

Martínez, E., Scoppetta, O., Castaño, G., Martín, A., & Pérez Gómez, A. (2019). The evaluation of a program in Colombia to prevent alcohol consumption. Learned Lessons. *Revista Argentina de Clinica Psicológica.*

Mejía, M. C. B., Toro, A. C., Espitia, J. A., Aristizábal, A. A., Echavarría, M. P., Trujillo, J. M., & Echavarría, A. (2018). Factores asociados al consumo de sustancias de abuso en pacientes embarazadas. Revista de la Facultad de Ciencias de la Salud Universidad del Cauca, 20(2), 22-28

Mejía-Trujillo, J., Pérez-Gómez, A., & Reyes-Rodríguez, M. (2015). Implementación y adaptación en Colombia del sistema preventivo Communities That Care. Adicciones, 27(4), 253-264. https://doi.org/10.20882/adicciones.750

Mejía-Trujillo, J. & Pérez-Gómez, A. (2023). Diez años de implementación del sistema preventivo Comunidades Que se Cuidan en Colombia. En Scoppetta-DG, O, Mejía-Trujillo, J. & Pérez-Gómez, A. (editores) (2023). Journal of Concurrent Disorders 5(3) 67-83. Special Issue.

Ministerio de Justicia y Dirección Nacional de Estupefacientes. (1996). OJO estudio pendiente. AUGUSTO lo envía

Ministerio de Justicia y del Derecho y Ministerio de Salud y Protección Social. (2014). Estudio de consumo de sustancias psicoactivas en población general. OJO AJUSTAR

Ministerio de Justicia y del Derecho - Observatorio de Drogas de Colombia, Ministerio de Educación Nacional y Ministerio de Salud y Protección Social. (2018), Estudio Nacional de consumo de sustancias psicoactivas en población escolar - Colombia 2016. Bogotá D.C. https://www.minjusticia.gov.co/programas-co/ODC/Publicaciones/Publicaciones/CO03142016_estudio_consumo_escolares_2016.pdf

Ministerio de Justicia y del Derecho - Observatorio de Drogas de Colombia, Instituto Colombiano de Bienestar Familiar (2017), Estudio de consumo de sustancias psicoactivas en el Sistema de Responsabilidad Penal Adolescente. Colombia 2017. Bogotá DC.: ODC.

Ministerio de Justicia y del Derecho – Observatorio de Drogas de Colombia (2019), Estudio Nacional de Consumo de Sustancias Psicoactivas Colombia 2019. Bogotá DC.: ODC.

Ministerio de Justicia y del Derecho – Observatorio de Drogas de Colombia, Ministerio de Educación Nacional (2022), Estudio Nacional de Consumo de Sustancias Psicoactivas Colombia en población escolar 2022. Bogotá DC.: ODC.

Ministerio de la Protección Social, UNODC, O. de las N. U. C. la D. y el D., RAISS Colombia, & Corporación Viviendo. (2009). *Modelo zonas de Orientación Escolar (ZOE).*

Montero-Zamora, P., Reyes-Rodríguez, M. F., Macías, F. C., Brown, E. C., Gómez, A. P., Trujillo, J. M., Bermúdez, J. T., & Aguilar, M. P. (2018). Uso de sustancias en adolescentes y su asociación con factores de riesgo y protección. Un análisis exploratorio de la encuesta escolar a gran escala de comunidades que se cuidan, Colombia. *Adicciones*, *32*(2), 105. https://doi.org/10.20882/adicciones.1083

Núñez, O., Ramírez-Vélez, R., & Correa-Bautista, J. E. (2019). Etapas de cambio comportamental frente al consumo de sustancias psicoactivas en escolares de 9 a 17 años de Bogotá D.C., Colombia. *Revista de la Facultad de Medicina*, *67*(1), 29-35. https://doi.org/10.15446/revfacmed.v67n1.65501

Oficina de las Naciones Unidas Contra la Droga & el Delito (UNODC) y el Ministerio de Justicia y del Derecho de Colombia. III Estudio epidemiológico andino sobre consumo de drogas en la población universitaria de Colombia., 2016.

Pedroza-Buitrago, A., Pulido-Reynel, A., Ardila-Sierra, A., Villa-Roel, S. M., González, P., Niño, L., & Piñeros, C. (2020). Consumo de alcohol, tabaco y sustancias psicoactivas de los adolescentes de un territorio indígena en la Amazonía colombiana. *Revista Colombiana de Psiquiatría*, *49*(4), 246-254. doi:https://doi.org/10.1016/j.rcp.2019.06.002

Pérez-Gómez, A., Cardozo-Macías, F. & Salcedo-Tocarruncho, L. Association Between Psychoactive Substance Abuse and Health Disorders in Colombian Problem Drug Users: Second Study. Int J Ment Health Addiction 18, 263–276 (2020). doi:https://doi.org/10.1007/s11469-018-9881-0

Pérez Gómez, A., Lanziano, C., Reyes Rodríguez, M. F., Mejía Trujillo, J., & Cardozo Macías, F. (2018). Perfiles asociados al consumo de alcohol en adolescentes colombianos. *Acta Colombiana de Psicología, 21*(2), 258–269. https://doi-org.ezproxy.uniminuto.edu/10.14718/acp.2018.21.2.12

Pérez-Gómez, A., & Scoppetta, O. (2015). Consumo de alcohol en menores de 18 años en Colombia: 2008. Estudio en siete capitales y dos municipios pequeños. Bogotá: CNR.

Pérez-Gómez, A., Mejía-Trujillo, J., Reyes-Rodríguez, M.F. & Cardozo, F. (2015). Consumo de alcohol en menores de 18 años en Colombia: 2015. Segundo estudio en siete capitales y dos municipios pequeños. Bogotá: CNR.

Pérez-Gómez, A., Mejía-Trujillo, J., Reyes-Rodríguez, M.F. & Cardozo, F. (2021). Consumo de alcohol en menores de 18 años en Colombia: 2021. Bogotá: CNR.

Pérez-Gómez, Villamil, A., Scoppetta, O., & Mejía-Trujillo, J. (2023). How much does it cost to the family for one of its members to be a drug and alcohol user. Journal of Concurrent Disorders. DOI: https://doi.org/10.54127/HVDO9867

Pineda Roa, C. A. (2015). Prevalencia y variables asociadas al consumo de sustancias psicoactivas en varones colombianos autoidentificados como homosexuales. Revista Iberoamericana de Psicología, 8(1), 83–91. https://doi.org/10.33881/2027-1786.rip.8108

Programa Presidencial Rumbos. (2002). Estudio nacional de consumo de drogas en jóvenes de 10 a 24 años. Bogotá: Presidencia de la República.

Ramírez, N., Díaz, M., Gantiva-Díaz, C. A., & Flórez-Alarcón, L. (2014). Del abuso de alcohol en escolares : análisis sistemático de dissemination of a procedure for the selective prevention of alcohol abuse in school : systematic case analysis. *Tipica Boletín electrónico de Salud Escolar, 10*(2).

Reyes-Rodríguez, M., Mejía-Trujillo, J., Pérez-Gómez, A., Cardozo, F., & Pinto, C. (2018) Effectiveness of a Brief Intervention based on Motivational Interviewing in Colombian Adolescents. Psicologia: Teoria e Pesquisa, 33, 1-7

Reyes-Rodríguez, M.F., Pinto-Gómez, J.C., Cardozo-Macías, F., Pérez-Gómez, A., Mejía-Trujillo, J., & Toro-Bermúdez, J. (2020). Evaluation of the prevention program "Brief Intervention based on Motivational Interviewing" in Colombian adolescents. Int J Ment Health Addiction 18 (2), 471-481. DOI https://doi.org/10.1007/s11469-019-0057-3

Riveros, F., Vera, L. A., Gantiva, C., & Torres, L. (2019). Adaptación del Cuestionario para Identificación de Trastornos Debidos al Consumo de Alcohol (AUDIT) en universitarios colombianos. Revista de Psicopatología y Psicología Clínica, 23(3), 231. doi:https://doi.org/10.5944/rppc.vol.23.num.3.2018.22258

Salcedo-Mejía, F., Alvis-Zakzuk, J., Paz-Wilches, J., Manrique-Mclean, J. P., Jeréz-Arias, M., & Alvis-Guzmán, N. (2018). Prevalencia y factores socioeconómicos asociados al consumo de alcohol en jóvenes de hogares pobres en la subregión Montes de María, en el Caribe colombiano. Revista Facultad Nacional de Salud Pública, 36(2), 37-48. https://doi.org/10.17533/udea.rfnsp.v36n2a06

Scoppetta, O., Anderson, P., Pérez-Gómez, A., Mejía-Trujillo, J., Solovei, A., O'Donnell, A. Jane-Llopis, E. & Rowlands, G. (2021). Feasibility of implementing Alcohol Health Literacy tests in Colombia. Journal of Alcohol and Drug Education (65)2: 61-85.

Scheuer, H., Kuklinski, M. R., Sterling, S. A., Catalano, R. F., Beck, A., Braciszewski, J., ... & Yoon, T. (2022). Parent-focused prevention of adolescent health risk behavior: Study protocol for a multisite cluster-randomized trial implemented in pediatric primary care. *Contemporary clinical trials, 112*, 106621.

Solovei, A., Manthey, J., Anderson, P., Mercken, L., Jané-Llopis, E., Natera, G., Pérez-Gómez, A., Mejía-Trujillo, J., Bustmante, I., Piazza, M., Pérez, A., Arroyo, M., de Vries, H., Rehm, J. & Evers, S. (2022). Costs of an Alcohol Measurement Intervention in Three Latin American Countries. International Journal of Environmental Research and Public Health doi:https://doi.org/10.3390/ijerph19020700

Augusto Pérez-Gómez obtained his PhD at Louvain's University (Belgium). He became Full Professor of Psychology at Los Andes University (Colombia), and a Visiting Professor at London University and the Robert Wood Johnson Medical School, University of Medicine and Dentistry of New Jersey; since 2002, he is the Director of Corporación Nuevos Rumbos, a non-profit organization dedicated to research and prevention of drug abuse and mental health problems. He has published 19 books and 236 papers (up to August 2025) in Spanish, English, French, German, and Portuguese (in that order).

Juliana Mejía-Trujillo is a social worker, with a Master's degree in Anthropology, PhD candidate at Maastricht University, the Netherlands. Currently, she works with Corporación Nuevos Rumbos as Director of Prevention. To date, she is the author and co-author of more than 70 publications (up to August 2025), including books, book chapters, and several articles in Spanish, English, and Portuguese.

Drug Abuse Prevention in Europe

Elisardo Becoña and Amador Calafat

Context

Europe is a continent located in the northern hemisphere where 747 million people live (448 in the European Union). It is washed by the Atlantic Ocean in the west, by the Mediterranean Sea, facing the African continent in the south, bordering Russia and Asia in the east, and the Arctic Ocean in the north. Although geographically Russia is part of Europe, it is considered separate, with its own entity, due to the enormous extension of that country, and its historical, cultural, and political characteristics. It currently has 146 million inhabitants. Communism emerged there in the last century as a political system, which it extended or imposed on other nearby European countries after World War II, in many cases by force. After the fall of the Berlin Wall and the subsequent social changes, these countries abandoned it, moved to a democratic system, and integrated into the economic (European Union) and political structures of Europe, with the exception of Russia, as it was considered a great power. It is currently at war with Ukraine, a neighboring country, which it wants to annex.

In Europe, what is known as Western culture was born, first in ancient Greece, then in Rome, which carried out the so-called Romanization of almost all of Europe, imposing a common language, Latin, as its homogeneous legal and political system, followed later throughout history by different wars, religious, cultural, political, and thought movements (e.g., the Renaissance, the Enlightenment). Hence the weight

E. Becoña (✉)
Universidad Santiago de Compostela, Santiago de Compostela, Spain
e-mail: elisardo.becona@usc.es

A. Calafat
Instituto Europeo de Estudios en Prevención – IREFREA, Palma de Mallorca, Spain

A. Pérez-Gómez, J. Mejía-Trujillo (eds.), *Drug Abuse Prevention*, Advances in Mental Health and Addiction, https://doi.org/10.1007/978-3-031-99621-4_4

that religion, politics, art, architecture, literature, thought, and science have had in the history of Europe.

Most European countries today make up the European Union (EU). Currently the EU is made up of 27 countries: Germany, Austria, Belgium, Bulgaria, Cyprus, Croatia, Denmark, Slovakia, Slovenia, Spain, Estonia, Finland, France, Greece, Hungary, Ireland, Italy, Latvia, Lithuania, Luxembourg, Malta, the Netherlands, Poland, Portugal, the Czech Republic, Romania, and Sweden, after the departure of the United Kingdom. Eight other countries are currently candidates for accession. Several countries are not integrated into it nor do they plan to do so, such as the United Kingdom, Switzerland, the Vatican, or other countries.

The EU is a common economic system, with equal political and social norms for all member states, which mark the economy, the political system, and part of its culture. The EU emerged after World War II. It is initially created by six countries (Germany, Belgium, France, Italy, Luxembourg, and the Netherlands) with the idea that greater integration between them will lead to replacing war with cooperation. The formula has been successful. Including the six initial countries there are now 27, and their number will continue to grow in the coming years. Although it is difficult for it to end up being a single state, cooperation between EU countries has been increasing year after year. Although they differ in language, culture, idiosyncrasy, history, or economy, their integration is a fact and has been successful, especially at an economic level, improving the living conditions of all countries, especially those that started from a worst level.

The economy of the European Union is the third in the world, after the United States and China, with a production of 15% of the world's total. Agriculture and fishing, industry, tourism, services, and energy have a great weight in its economy. It exports many of its products, and some countries are world leaders in their industry. Several of them have the highest GDPs in the world.

Europe is known by the so-called welfare state. As an example, all countries make a strong public investment in health, education, and research, with access to health and education being free for all, or almost free, financed through taxes. There is a clear social redistribution of wealth. The same goes for retirement, with an adequate living allowance, and other social rights and advantages for the most disadvantaged. It has a good system of social services for people without resources.

Currently, the majority of the population is between 30 and 50 years old, with a high percentage of older people in southern Europe, due to their high life expectancy. The progressive aging of the population, due to the low birth rate that has been dragging on since the 1980s, means that there is a smaller youth population. This has led to significant immigration, especially from North Africa, as well as from Latin American (LA) countries and the EU itself, from Western countries to those in Central Europe, because the latter have more resources and need for labor.

The two predominant religions are Catholic, especially in the south, and Protestant, in the center and north. Orthodox or Muslim predominates in some western countries. They are practiced, but as a minority, Jewish and others in different countries. A percentage of the population is non-believer, about a quarter of it.

A large number of languages are spoken in Europe. The predominant ones are German, English, French, Spanish, Italian, and Greek. Some countries have several official languages.

Introduction

Europe is a continent where 747 million people currently live. Most countries make up the European Union (EU). Currently the EU is made up (2023) of 27 countries: Germany, Austria, Belgium, Bulgaria, Cyprus, Croatia, Denmark, Slovakia, Slovenia, Spain, Estonia, Finland, France, Greece, Hungary, Ireland, Italy, Latvia, Lithuania, Luxembourg, Malta, the Netherlands, Poland, Portugal, the Czech Republic, Romania, and Sweden, after the departure of the United Kingdom. Eight other countries are currently candidates for accession. The epidemiological data of the European Monitoring Center for Drugs and Drug Addiction (EMCDDA) includes data from member states, along with Norway, a European country that is not a member of the EU, although it has been linked to it for decades through the European Economic Area (EEA). It also usually includes data on candidates to join the EU.

The EU is largely the result of World War II. It was initially created by six countries (Germany, Belgium, France, Italy, Luxembourg, and the Netherlands) with the idea that greater integration between them will lead to replacing war with cooperation. The formula has been successful because including those initial six countries there are now 27. Although it is difficult for it to end up being a single state, cooperation between EU countries has been increasing year after year. Although they differ in language, culture, idiosyncrasy, history, economy, their integration is a fact and has been successful, especially at an economic level, improving the living conditions of all European countries, especially those that started from a worst level. All EU countries have a drug policy. All information is monitored by the European Monitoring Center for Drugs and Drug Addiction (EMCDDA), whose headquarters are in Lisbon (Portugal). This allows us to know the problem, what is being done today, and what can be improved. That is why there is talk of the "European Union model" in drugs (Culley et al. 2012).

Drug consumption in Europe is very relevant, one of the highest in the world, especially marijuana, the main illegal drug consumed, along with cocaine and heroin. Many European countries suffered from the heroin epidemic in the 1970s and 1980s. In recent years we have experienced the cocaine epidemic and, in the coming years, that of marijuana (Rödner et al. 2008).

As we have already pointed out, within the EU there is a specific agency on the problem of illegal drug consumption. It prepares different studies on preventive measures, treatment, and social reintegration. On the EMCDDA website you can publicly access its reports, publications, and multiple information on drugs (www.emcdda.europa.eu). In addition, this page is in all EU languages, including Spanish.

By reviewing the multiple information it contains, you can get a good idea of the state of affairs regarding drugs in Europe and its member states.

Treatment remains the predominant field in all countries, but much work has also been done in the preventive field. This has been necessary due to the high incidence and prevalence of drug use in its different countries. Some of the drugs consumed in the EU come from other countries or continents, as is the case with hashish (the hashish resin obtained from marijuana) coming mainly from Morocco, a country located opposite Spain on the African continent; cocaine from Latin America, produced mainly in Bolivia, Colombia, and Peru, and introduced from different countries to Europe by sea and air (e.g., from Colombia, Brazil, Venezuela, among other countries); heroin from Afghanistan mainly and to a lesser extent Iran and Pakistan. As for synthetic drugs, they began to be manufactured in Eastern European countries; at the moment they are produced within the EU. Europe has also become a major producer of marijuana, especially for domestic consumption.

Thanks to the EMCDDA, all European countries have at least one focal point (within the REITOX network; EU Drugs Agency Information on Drugs and Drug Addiction) and most have created their own National Observatory or National Plan to study the drug phenomenon and coordinate different preventive and therapeutic measures. This has made it easier to implement measures such as conducting epidemiological studies on drug use, opening treatment centers for addicts or including them in the health system, and implementing preventive measures at school to reduce drug use. In practice, the measures that have been implemented the most have been those related to treatment, which were initially fundamentally psychological, and in recent years we have had more medical ones as different drugs have become available for treatment, especially methadone for heroin, or for the treatment of comorbidity so linked to them. Prevention has always had its importance in Europe, but it has been established irregularly and is more subject to political and economic fluctuations. In recent years, great importance has been given to evaluating preventive programs, providing evidence-based prevention, and disseminating both good preventive programs and good prevention practices (UNODOC 2013, 2018).

The truth is that we can speak of a European model on drugs, as we will see later, which is different from those that exist in the United States and Latin American countries. There is, however, a variety of situations, from those countries with more traditional policies where the emphasis is on control, to those in which the emphasis is on harm reduction, although there is a movement of many states to give more weight on harm reduction. Although prevention and harm reduction are not opposite paradigms, but rather completely complementary, it is a fact that the development of harm reduction policies is sometimes done to the detriment of typically preventive programs. In Europe, capital movements are controlled to prevent money laundering from drug trafficking. There is also important coordination for the control of precursors and police euro warrants to the control of crime due to drug trafficking, which occurs in all European countries, greater cross-border cooperation between countries to prosecute these crimes, etc.

There is also great concern about the appearance of new drugs, especially synthetic ones, which are becoming more numerous every year, and the sale of drugs through the Internet, as is the current example of synthetic cathinones.

Evolution of Public Policies and Their Current State

Epidemiology of Drug Use in Europe

In Europe, different EU countries systematically carry out surveys of the general and/or school population to find out the prevalence of drug use. These surveys are included in the annual report of the European Monitoring Center for Drugs and Drug Addiction (EMCDDA). In this way we know year by year the prevalence of consumption. At the same time, we have a large survey carried out periodically among children and young people in school, which is the ESPAD project (European School Survey Project on Alcohol and Other Drugs), from 1995 to the present, with 39 countries currently participating (www.espad.org) (ESPAD Group 2020). Also, for this population, different European countries carry out their own surveys. Spain is one of the countries that has an uninterrupted series of representative surveys of the general population (EDADES survey) and schoolchildren (ESTUDES survey) and which can be consulted on the website of the National Plan on Drugs (www.pnsd.sanidad.gob. is). There are other EU organizations that also carry out studies to find out different aspects, opinions, beliefs, and attitudes about drug consumption, such as the Eurobarometers on illicit drugs that have been carried out since 2002 (European Commission 2022). There are also Eurobarometers on alcohol and tobacco.

The 2022 EMCDDA report has been prepared with the information provided by the various national reports of the EU member states, the candidate country Turkey, as well as Norway. In relation to substances, the report focuses on the main ones, such as cannabis, opiates, and stimulants. The report does not include tobacco or alcohol. These data are kept by offices other than the EU, although the consumption of these substances at a preventive level will later have great relevance.

In relation to cannabis, the report indicates the polarization that exists today in Europe in opinion polls about it and the important public debate in some countries, but not all, about the substance, especially aimed at recreational consumption. Most allow the medical use of cannabis or cannabinoids. As the report says, the consumption situation is "complex." Significant consumption has been reached, probably at the top, with new synthetic cannabinoid products emerging, with a very dynamic market. In the years of Covid-19 confinement there has been a decrease in consumption. The increase in cannabis production in recent years in many European countries stands out. The average tetrahidrocannabinol (THC) content has increased greatly (21% for hashish resin, 11% for marijuana, and up to 35% with new types of marijuana). There is concern about the increase in synthetic cannabinoids. In

Europe as a whole, cannabis is now the main drug most frequently reported as the first request for treatment for illegal drugs. Cannabis seizures in Europe are very important, around half of all those made for illegal drugs (specifically, the 2022 report indicates 584 tons of hashish and 155 tons of herb (marijuana) of the total seized in Europe, with the majority in Spain, as it is the country of entry from Morocco to Europe for this drug). To give us a comparative idea, the heroin seized in Europe was 5 tons, and 213 tons of cocaine.

An important entry point for heroin is Turkey. Furthermore, in the Baltic countries around Turkey, heroin is being replaced by other substances, in particular synthetic opioids and stimulants. The positive thing is that heroin overdoses have decreased. But, in some countries such as Estonia, an increase in deaths from the use of synthetic opioids has been reported, which has been linked to the use of fentanyls, a family of very powerful synthetic opioids. Furthermore, the majority of deaths occur in polydrug abusers, which indicates a significant level of severity in addiction. The 2022 report indicates that 3.5 tons, 130 liters, and 1.6 million synthetic opioid tablets were seized.

In relation to stimulants, cocaine continues to be the preferred stimulant in southern and western countries, with amphetamine predominating in northern and eastern countries. The increase in methamphetamine production in Central Europe, as well as its consumption, also stands out. A similar increase occurs with ecstasy (or MDMA), which is mainly manufactured in Belgium and the Netherlands. In 2020, 4.7 million ecstasy pills were seized in Europe. Different derivatives of cathinones (e.g., mephedrone) also spread throughout Europe. Likewise, new psychoactive substances continue to appear, produced in Europe or imported from China or India. Another problem that is more frequently observed is the use of different medications as drugs, especially in opiate users (e.g., pregabalin, phenazepam, diazepam, phenibut). The consumption of other drugs such as hallucinogens, GHB (gamma-hydroxybutyrate), and ketamine is low and stable.

But despite everything said, the cost of treatment is predominantly based on problems derived from the heroin epidemic of past decades. It is the drug that produces the greatest morbidity and mortality (e.g., due to overdose). Since heroin dependence is one of the most chronic disorders, and with many associated chronic diseases (HIV, hepatitis C, etc.), it requires dedicating many therapeutic resources to it. For example, the latest estimate for Europe is that there are currently around 514,000 people in treatment with opiate substitutes out of the million problem heroin users that exist. Parenteral consumption has also decreased. Many of the national drug plans or observatories of European countries were created precisely to confront the heroin epidemic. Luckily, the demands for treatment for this substance are decreasing. The negative aspect of the data is that demands for treatment with other opiates such as methadone, buprenorphine, and fentanyl are increasing.

Drug consumption, at the prevalence level, both following the ESPAD survey, in school children, and the data from the different countries in their national surveys, are indicated synthetically in Table 1. There are important differences between countries, but these data allow us to see the trends and prevalence of drugs consumed in Europe.

Table 1 Estimates of drug consumption in the European Union, people aged 15–65 and 15–34 years

	People from 15 to 65 years old		Young people from 15 to 34 years old	
Substance	Life	Past-year	Past-year	Rank by country
Cannabis	27.3%	7.7%	15.5%	1.8–21.8
Cocaine	5.0%	1.2%	2.2%	0.2–4.6
Amphetamines	3.1%	0.7%	1.4%	0.0–4.1
Ecstasy	3.7%	0.9%	1.9%	0.2–8.5

The EMCDDA's 2023 interim report (2023) is along the same lines as what we have just discussed.

As the 2014 EMCDDA Report rightly said: "the global situation remains generally stable, with positive signs in some areas, but new challenges continue to appear. The old dichotomy between a relatively small number of highly problematic, often injecting, drug users, and a larger number of recreational and experimental users is breaking down and being replaced by a more gradual and complex situation. In the field of drug addiction in Europe, heroin plays a less relevant role today than in the past, while stimulants, synthetic drugs, cannabis and medicines are becoming increasingly important".

But, along with these "classic" drugs with well-known effects and consequences, there has been growing concern for years about the appearance of new substances. In recent years, a large number of new substances have been identified for the first time in Europe through the Rapid Detection System which is controlled by the EMCDDA and Europol. Specifically, there are currently 880 new substances under study. According to the EMCDDA, they have a varied chemical composition (cathinones, cannabinoids, phenylethylamines, opioids, etc.). In 2020, 7 tons of these substances were seized (almost half cathinone powder). Along with these substances are "legal highs," which contain psychoactive substances that have not normally been banned, and which are sold mainly in so-called smart shops, which are stores that sell seeds or plants that do not have psychoactive properties, but once planted and cultivated, psychoactive substances are obtained (e.g., marijuana, hallucinogenic mushrooms). Along with the appearance of these substances, there is also the problem of new sales and distribution systems through the Internet, which are reaching great expansion and which are very complicated to control, door-to-door distribution, etc. On the other hand, the consumption of hallucinogenic and dissociative drugs is low in Europe.

Two facts that must be commented on, and that have great relevance today, and may have more relevance in the future. The first is the fall of Afghanistan into the hands of the Taliban. Afghanistan is the leading producer of opium in the world, over 85% of the total, with an important part of the country's economy depending on it. This can lead to a greater increase in the availability of opium given the situation in which that country finds itself. The second is the invasion of part of Ukraine by Russia. This changes some drug entry routes into Europe. The consequences of war can directly affect drug consumption in the medium term.

European Drug Policy

There is a trend towards homogenization of the forms of consumption and abuse of the various legal and illegal drugs in Europe. Policies are also converging more and more, but in practice, especially if we think about their real application, there are still differences (e.g., between eastern European countries and western ones and also between Scandinavian countries—Sweden, Norway—and those from southern Europe). The Nordic countries are the ones that have most effectively applied preventive health policies for decades (and not only on drug issues) (Mackenbach and McKee 2013).

We must keep in mind that drug policies are basically a matter that depends on the will of each country. One of the paradigmatic examples is tobacco, with respect to which some countries have taken clear actions, while for others they considered it an issue that depends on individual responsibility. In the case of alcohol, the Scandinavian countries have a history of temperance movements dating back to the nineteenth century and which have meant limited access to alcohol (through state monopolies) and high taxes. These policies have been limited by the entry of these countries into the European Union where antitrust laws exist.

There is a European Strategic Plan on drugs that is renewed periodically (the latest is from 2021–2025). The priorities are the usual ones. It is about promoting access and application of evidence-based programs, promoting the implementation of standards in prevention and harm reduction. Special emphasis is placed on new challenges such as consumers who use various drugs at the same time (many times also legal and illegal), the illegal use of drugs, also the use of new psychoactive substances and Internet sales.

The EU drug strategy is based on a public health approach. It gives relevance to legal and illegal drugs, as well as the consumption of non-prescription medications, due to their abuse (whether obtained with or without a medical prescription). Note the strong pressure that exists from the pharmaceutical industry in developed countries to medicalize the entire population (Gotzsche 2014; Frances 2014).

The EU Drugs Strategy 2021–2025 has recently been approved (see:https://www.consilium.europa.eu/media/54074/qc0521073esn_002.pdf), which continues as the previous ones. It outlines the lines and actions to follow in these years, through six axes: reduction of drug supply; drug demand reduction; addressing drug-related harm; international cooperation; research, innovation, and foresight; and, coordination, governance, and application. From these the guidelines of the different national drug plans are obtained.

This Strategic Plan (e.g., the current one for 2021–2025) is accompanied by a more specific "Action Plan" which insists on common needs such as basing drug policies on powerful scientific evidence at the European level, although later in practice, specific funding sources for drug issues have been disappearing. Another handicap is that there are few powers at the European level to demand these policies, which basically depend on the will of each member state. Its role is above all to coordinate and avoid duplication, promote cooperation, and ensure that the objectives are assumed by the member states. But it is the responsibility of each member state to adopt the legal frameworks, strategies, budgets, type of organization, the relevance of prevention, etc. In practice—although there is a tendency towards homogenization—this implies notable differences in the legislation and penalties for personal drug consumption, drug trafficking, money laundering, etc.

One of the key pillars of this entire European strategy is the specific agency created to address illegal drugs: the European Monitoring Centre for Drugs and Drug Addiction (EMCDDA), which, as mentioned above, is located in Lisbon, Portugal. This agency is key, among other things, in collecting data at the European level, promoting the homogenization of policies and information collection, studying new problems or managing the European drug information network made up of a series of national focal points called REITOX. The EMCDDA produces an annual report on the situation of illegal drugs in Europe and offers a series of publications that can be obtained on its website www.emcdda.europa.eu.

There are other European organizations that have to do with policies and actions in relation to illegal drugs, such as European Union Agency for Law Enforcement Cooperation (EUROPOL) (the body that coordinates police actions at European level) and the Horizontal Group on Drugs, which is a group of representatives of the member countries that meet frequently to monitor the situation.

One of the initiatives that helps frame prevention in Europe is the publication of standards for preventive programs (European Monitoring Centre for Drugs and Drug Addiction [EMCDDA] 2011), which defines the basic and professional criteria for carrying out prevention in Europe. The manual covers all phases of building and implementing a program (design, implementation, evaluation, dissemination, etc.).

Regarding alcohol, there is a common tax scheme regulated by a European Union Directive (a rule that once approved by the European Parliament has to be transposed into the legislation of each EU country), which in theory should allow taxation to be used with preventive intent. But in practice there are large discrepancies and, for example, in the Nordic countries the tax is applied proportionally to the amount of alcohol in each drink, something that does not happen in other countries such as wine producers, where products such as wine or beer tends to be seen as food products (Villalbí et al. 2014).

In recent years, the weight that has been given in Europe, as in other countries, to environmental prevention stands out (Becoña 2021; Burkhart 2011; Oncioiu et al. 2018), an effective way to reduce consumption through laws and regulations implemented in each country. It is one of the preventive ways with the greatest future in the coming years.

National Drug Policies in Europe

As we have already indicated, although there is a European strategy on drugs, the importance of each European country is decisive in legal issues, pointing out their priorities, specifying their budgets, etc. The European strategy can indicate priorities and facilitate coordination, but everything else depends exclusively on each member state. While it is true that there is a tendency towards homogenization (e.g., penalizing those who offer drugs more than the consumers themselves), this is not always the case.

All states (with the exception of Austria, which has regional plans instead of a national strategy) have a strategy on illegal drugs. But, while in a series of states there is a joint strategy for legal and illegal drugs (which coincides with the fact that in practice such consumption is closely linked), others maintain separate strategies. Recently, several European states have adopted, with notable success, specific laws on tobacco consumption in public places (for more details you can consult the EMCDDA's annual report on the European situation www.emcdda.europa.eu). A very direct way to know the degree of involvement of the states in the drug problem is to look at the public spending allocated specifically to these matters. Although making comparisons is sometimes difficult due to the way in which the data is presented (and the administrative complexity of each country), we find some countries spend a notable amount (such as Croatia, Sweden, or the Netherlands), compared to others with smaller investments (France, Portugal, or Italy) (United Nations 2007).

One of the characteristics of the current situation is the growing importance of civil society in drug matters. There is a European mandate by which the opinion of civil society must be sought, which is why the Civil Society Forum on Drugs has been established a few years ago (www.civilsocietyforumondrugs.eu). But the most characteristic thing, for a few years now, is the appearance and growing activity of civil associations (more than 200 according to a recent EMCDDA study) that are active especially in issues of legalization or harm reduction. Their activity sometimes leads to detracting from other actions such as prevention.

A specific analysis for each country can be found on the EMCDDA website: https://www.emcdda.europa.eu/countries_en.

Prevention Actions

Preventive Programs at European Level

In recent decades, a large number of preventive programs have been developed in different EU countries. Also, programs from other countries (especially North America) have been investigated in different European countries to verify their proper functioning in different contexts and cultures.

In Europe, as in the Anglo-Saxon world, there is great concern for evidence based treatment and prevention. In the preventive field, this is understood as the use of scientific results to inform intervention decisions in the areas of prevention, treatment, and harm reduction in drug use (Ferri and Bo 2013).

In 2002 the EMCDDA created a web portal of good practices for: (1) interventions in demand reduction, (2) European prevention, treatment, harm reduction, and social integration projects, (3) an inventory of good practice standards including a bank of instruments to evaluate interventions. All of this can be consulted electronically at www.emcdda.europa.eu/best-practice. All the selection of the above has been done following the methods of the Cochrane Collaboration, which is also available in Spanish (www.cochrane.es). In short, for the EMCDDA "best practice is the best application of the evaluation of the available evidence in the field of drugs." Faced with the ideal of evidence-based programs, reality also forces us to give a place to programs that we consider "good practices."

The objective of the EMCDDA portal is to disseminate best practices in the field of drugs. The website allows access to all that information. And, at the same time, as it is available, countries should implement best practices. Within the portal, the EDDRA (The Exchange on Drug Demand Reduction) network stands out, which is a database within the good practice portal that provides concrete examples of programs that meet the good practice requirements that are being carried out in different EU countries. Any person, institution, or country can submit a proposal to be included in EDDRA. A committee of experts will evaluate it and if it considers that it meets the requirements of good practices, it will be included. Within the prevention section, four sections are considered: family, school students, community members, and general population. The portal's evidence classification is: beneficial, probably beneficial, neither beneficial nor harmful; we do not know the effectiveness and evidence of ineffectiveness.

The EDDRA good practices portal currently includes modules on prevention, treatment, harm reduction, and social reintegration. Currently this database includes 500 projects; of these, 270 are prevention programs from different European countries (in Table 2 we indicate the Spanish preventive programs that appear there, as in the most recent one from Xchange, also from the EMCDDA).

Examples of Representative Programs at European Level

We have several examples of preventive programs that have been implemented in different European countries. We are going to focus on two of them: Unplugged and Up to you.

The Unplugged program has been carried out within the study called EU-Dap. This program was evaluated through a randomized cluster study, with an experimental and control group (who received the usual curriculum) and an 18-month follow-up. It is a universal preventive program, applied at school, for children between 12 and 14 years of age. One hundred and seventy schools from seven

Table 2 Spanish preventive programs included in the EDDRA network and in the EMCDDA's Xchange, with different levels of effectiveness and usefulness

EDDRA:
– Family competition program. University of the Balearic Islands, Palma de Mallorca
– Brief intervention in alcohol-related traffic injuries. Prevention and Care Service for Dependencies. Barcelona Public Health Agency
– "You decide" program. Irefrea. Palma de Mallorca
Xchange:
– Unplugged program
– Life Skills Training Program
– Let's Get Started Program
– TAKE CARE
– Program You decide
– EQUIPMENT
– About Cannabis and Joints

countries participated (Germany, Austria, Belgium, Spain, Greece, Italy, and Sweden) with a total of 7079 participants. The program consists of 12 one-hour interactive sessions, applied by teachers (Vigna-Taglianti et al. 2014). The evaluation was done through an anonymous questionnaire self-completed by each student in the pre-, post-intervention and follow-ups up to 18 months after the application of the program. Both the program and the questionnaire have been the same in the different countries, with their respective translations.

This program is based on the theory of social learning, the theory of problem behavior, the health belief model, the theory of reasoned action and planned behavior, and the theory of social norms (Vadrucci et al. 2016). A description of them can be seen in Becoña (1999, 2002). Its components include training in creative and critical thinking, decision-making, problem-solving, effective communication, interpersonal relationship skills, self-awareness, empathy, coping with emotions and stress, normative beliefs, and knowledge about the harmful consequences of drugs (Van der Kreeft et al. 2009).

The results indicated at 3 months of follow-up that this program was more effective than the control group in preventing tobacco and cannabis use, as well as in reducing the frequency of binge drinking (e.g., 3.9% binge drinking in the control group and 2.5% in the experimental group) (Faggiano et al. 2008; Giannotta et al. 2014).

After 18 months of follow-up, the program Unplugged is significantly more effective than the control in reducing any binge drinking, frequent binge drinking, and frequent cannabis use. No effects appear for tobacco consumption, losing the effect that existed after 3 months of follow-up. They found differences by sex, with men being the ones who consume more, specifically tobacco daily, episodes of drunkenness, and cannabis consumption.

Another important result of the study is that the preventive program has an important effect on people from low socioeconomic levels, a fact of great relevance because it prevents drug consumption (Vigna-Taglianti et al. 2014) and, with it, different effects, unwanted consequences that usually accompany it, such as lower academic performance or premature abandonment of school. For example, people from low socioeconomic levels started with higher alcohol consumption, with the preventive program decreasing the episodes of drunkenness (Odds Ratio, OR = 0.60), intention to get drunk (OR = 0.60), and problem behaviors related to alcohol (OR = 0.70) (Caria et al. 2011a, b).

In another study with this same program, to know the factors that mediate the effectiveness of the program, they found three: attitudes, rejection skills, and the perception of prevention of drug use among peers (Giannotta et al. 2014).

The program Up to you is a universal school preventive program designed in Spain in 1985 (Calafat et al. 1985) by members of the current team of Irefrea, one of the main European associations dedicated to prevention (www.irefrea.org). It is the first Spanish program to be evaluated and its design is carried out after having implemented and evaluated a first prototype. The program has undergone various adaptations, sometimes more formal (such as changing the design of the comic strip characters) and sometimes more in-depth, such as adding some modules (in the 2008 and 2023 versions; Calafat et al. 2008a, 2023): one on Internet use and the other on the relationship with parents, in the 2008 version. Throughout 2022 and 2023, considerable work has been done to achieve a version that can be applied online with European Funds. Within this same year, the evaluation of this online version begins. It is a program taught in principle by the teachers themselves (although it has also been done with experts from outside the school) and it also has a module that involves families based on calls made by the teacher himself.

The program consists of some comics (with some characters that are repeated and that present typical situations in which decisions must be made, but without the meaning of the decision being resolved within the story) with some additional information. But the key to the program are the sessions that are organized during class time (normally between 6 and 10, although they can be more) starting with the reading of the comics and then normally entering into various interactive dynamics, where the role of "active neutrality" from the teacher is absolutely key.

There are two experimental evaluations with a control group, one carried out by the team itself (Calafat et al. 1989) and the other by a team from the University of Barcelona (1989–1992). There is currently another one underway, as we have already said about the online version, the results of which will be known soon. The results show that there are fewer drinkers and lower consumption after 2 years within the experimental group compared to the control group, and there are also fewer people who start smoking. Furthermore, there are several qualitative evaluations or evaluations on partial aspects of the methodology used (Kornblit et al. 1990; Macià et al. 1993).

In 1995 it was a widely followed program in Spain with more than 12,000 students in different places such as Barcelona, Mallorca, Zaragoza, Jaca, Reus, and Vigo. It has been incorporated in recent years in various places in Portugal such as the Azores Islands, where it became the official program. According to the process evaluation carried out in 1984 by Rodríguez-Martos et al. (1996), its good acceptance by teachers and students stands out. Teachers use the proposed interactive techniques, but there is more difficulty in using those that involve dramatization. It is noted how teachers quickly identify with the program despite the fact that the training they have followed on it is sometimes limited and how the program has managed to expand without there being a centralized structure that promotes it (Calafat et al. 2023).

The program is included with very good ratings both on the Spanish portal www.prevencionbasadaenlaevidencia.net as in the European portal EDDRA and Xchange of the EMCDDA in Lisbon (www.emcdda.europa.eu).

"Evidence-Based Prevention" Platforms

Making prevention based on evidence has become a priority assumed by prevention for a long time, just as it is already common in other fields such as treatment. But in practice, both in Europe and elsewhere, many programs currently being implemented have not been evaluated or this evaluation has not been rigorous enough to determine that we are dealing with an evidence-based program. Without this having to serve as an excuse for not making the necessary efforts to have a catalog of evidence-based programs, we do have to confirm that evaluating prevention represents important challenges as drug consumption is a changing field, as it is difficult sometimes to get adequate control groups etc. (National Academies of Sciences, Engineering, and Medicine [NASEM] 2019; O'Connell et al. 2009).

We have already mentioned that the European Commission's strategy supports this orientation and that quality standards in prevention have been promoted (EMCDDA 2011). Also various international organizations Comisión Interamericana para el Control del Abuso de Drogas (CICAD), Cooperation Program between Latin America, the Caribbean and the European Union on drug policy (COPOLAD), National Institute on Drug Abuse (NIDA), United Nations Office on Drugs and Crime (UNODOC) would be within the same strategic vision. However, there is still a lack of an initiative at the European level that de facto brings together this initiative. The powers at European level are basically to set priorities and facilitate coordination, but decisions and actions continue to depend on national levels. Therefore, there is no regulatory framework for the implementation of preventive programs at the European level and, in general, not at the level of the member countries themselves. It would be important to advance a policy that regulates this situation and prioritizes public funding towards programs that have proven effective, or towards their research.

There are several national initiatives (e.g., the German one: www.gruene-liste-praevention.de/nano.cms/datenbank/information) that clearly meet this objective of collecting and analyzing the preventive programs used in the respective countries. The evaluations that support it are studied for each program and finally an assessment is issued on the quality of such evidence, which is expressed in the form of a number of stars. The maximum number of stars is awarded to well-constructed programs whose application gives positive results after having been subjected to one (or several) external evaluation, with the widest possible follow-up.

In the Netherlands we also find similar initiatives supported by the government and carried out by two organizations (Centers for Healthy Living and Youth Health of the National Institute for Public Health and the Environment and the Netherlands Youth Institute).

In Spain we have two of these initiatives: Evidence-Based Prevention (www.prevencionbasadaenlaevidencia.net) and the Portal of Good Practices in Drug Demand Reduction (RDD).

The Spanish platform on Evidence-Based Prevention began in 2011 with support from Spain's National Drug Plan. We began by creating a scientific committee of six professionals, all of them experts in prevention and with editorial experience (very useful in this case as it is a skill that helps review and make decisions). A committee of experts was also established that included a large majority of professionals active in prevention in Spain, with significant experience, so that they could serve as reviewers, provide their comments, send programs, etc. The next step consisted of identifying, through various sources, the various existing programs that were active, that were not specific activities, and that had a certain entity to be considered programs. Seventy programs were identified, of which 51 were finally included for evaluation. No program rated by the platform received the maximum score of four stars (normally because despite being able to demonstrate good results, there was no external evaluation). But there were four that got three stars, all of them referring to the school environment (Building health; About Canyes i petes; BCN Pass; Up to you). The evaluation method used is quasi-experimental with intervention and control group, with follow-up, etc. All have internal evaluation, except "Up to you," which also offers another by an external team. The platform also offers a selection of articles, guides, and technical aids for research and evaluation, which facilitate the work of researchers.

The Portal of Good Practices in Drug Demand Reduction (RDD) is a collaborative project between the Autonomous Community of the Region of Murcia and the Government Delegation for the National Plan on Drugs, with the collaboration of the Autonomous Plans on Drugs, the Spanish Federation of Municipalities and Provinces (FEMP), the European Observatory on Drugs and Drug Addiction (EMCDDA) and COPOLAD (www.buenaspracticasadicciones.es/).

The European Society for Prevention Research (EUSPR)

In 2011, the European Society for Prevention Research was created at the European level (European Society for Prevention Research-EUSPR, www.euspr.org). It was inspired by the North American Society of Prevention Research. As its statutes state, its mission is to advance the science of environmentally based, universal, selective, and indicated prevention with the goal of improving human health, well-being, and reducing health inequalities. For this society, interdisciplinarity among scientists, developing public policies, developing methodologies, and promoting greater education and professional development in prevention and the implementation of research are basic elements.

The emergence of this organization is due to the need to have a scientific society dedicated to prevention at the European level given that there is a large number of professionals who work in this field, but little interconnected with each other, the development of a large number of preventive programs, the good evaluation of different preventive programs at the European level, and the need to join efforts at the European level to work as a network. Although the society has a generic title of prevention, in practice almost all the professionals that form it are from the field of drug prevention—possibly because it is the field where there is greater tradition and experience, but also includes professionals from public health, epidemiology, medicine, psychology, and other sciences. Its current members come from almost all European countries. It holds an annual conference that allows the exchange of scientific information, learning of new prevention research methodologies, learning about new preventive programs, and facilitating knowledge among its members to be able to participate in European projects that are convened annually to be carried out by professionals and institutions from several European countries. The society also admits members from other countries. Likewise, it has good coordination in various initiatives of the European Monitoring Center for Drugs and Drug Addiction in Lisbon, universities, and other scientific associations in the field of prevention in other European countries and the United States.

Prevention Networks in Europe

A notable aspect of the EU in relation to other countries is the financing of different European projects and networks in the field of drugs, including prevention. They have to be made up of people from different countries. This allows for important collaboration between countries and researchers, with different points of view, delimiting what is scientific from what is not, seeing the peculiarities of each country reflected in the work to be done, making known and merging different and/or complementary experiences, establish fluid relationships between people and researchers, and, with all this, reach common standards or procedures. The result is being excellent in most of them. Thanks to them, it is really possible for all Europeans to know each other better, to collaborate in the common task, to know how to share different points of view, to open our minds to new ideas, to network (of people, via email, other electronic resources, and to have own websites), learn first-hand about the level of research and technological development of each country, as well as its level of economic and social development, how its lifestyle is organized, and get to know different European countries and cities in coordination meetings, conferences, congresses, etc.

English is the language of intercommunication between them. This is a handicap for those countries that do not prioritize this language, especially those in southern

Europe. In addition, there are other common elements, such as the single currency (euro) in all its countries, a similar economy with common European guidelines (e.g., through the European Central Bank and the Eurogroup), without physical borders, with freedom of movement between countries—for people, goods and services—with a mobility program for students and teachers (the Erasmus Programme), or having the European higher education area in all countries to exchange students and qualifications for equivalence (the educational model of Bologna).

We are going to illustrate the above with two examples, with a network specifically dedicated to prevention throughout Europe (Irefrea) and another network that focused in previous years more on research and teaching (the European SPAN (Science for Prevention Academic Network) project).

- The Irefrea network (European Institute for Prevention Studies)

The Irefrea network (www.irefrea.org) was founded in 1988 with prevention experts from several European countries. It is the oldest professional network in the field of drug prevention in Europe. The Spanish group maintains the scientific leadership of the different research projects developed since the group's inception. Areas covered by Irefrea include research, implementation, and evaluation of programs on issues such as alcohol and other drug use and related risk factors. The Irefrea network is an international reference in topics such as recreational prevention, with multiple research and interventions. In this field it has developed standards (Calafat et al. 2012), designed training courses, organized conferences, etc. The network has also been active in developing the "You decide" school program (Calafat et al. 1985, 2008a, b, 2023), which as previously stated has been widely used in Spain and Portugal (and included with good evaluation in both EDDRA and on the Spanish platform "prevenciónbasadaenlaevidencia.net") and the family empowerment program Familias en Red y Activas (FERYA) (www.ferya.es) (Juan et al. 2018).

IREFREA (European Institute for Prevention Studies) members are very active in various professional and scientific fields, and regularly collaborate with organizations such as the European Monitoring Center for Drugs and Drug Addiction (EMCDDA), the European Community, the National Institute on Drug Abuse (NIDA), the United Nations Office on Drugs and Crime (UNODC) and the Government Delegation for the National Plan on Drugs (PNSD); in addition to actively participating in networks such as EuroCare, the European Society for Prevention Research, the European Civil Society Forum on Drugs, and the Club-Health initiative. He has made a good number of publications, which can be seen on his website (www.irefrea.org and www.irefrea.eu).

- The SPAN project

In the SPAN (Science for Prevention Academic Network) project (https://euspr.org/science-for-prevention-academic-network-span/) 32 groups from 15 European countries (about 100 people) participated with the aim of knowing the state of prevention in Europe, both in the professional and academic fields, to, based on said analysis, make concrete proposals. The project began in 2013 and ended in 2017. It was coordinated from Oxford Brookes University, in the United Kingdom.

In this case, as in others, although it is oriented towards all aspects of prevention, in practice it ends up focusing on the field of drug prevention, because this field is the place where the most professionals work in each country. Great importance was given to multidisciplinarity and collaborative networking, with professionals in the preventive field, specialists in research methodology, academics, etc.

European projects are structured, apart from the leader who will coordinate all the actions of the project, into specific actions of the same, which are called Work Packages (WP). Each project has several WPs, with a leader of each WP and several participants in it, while group members usually participate in more than one WP, thus achieving transversality and integration. The following WPs are included in the SPAN project: program coordination, dissemination and communication of results, knowledge of tertiary prevention science education and training in Europe, analysis of prevention workforce needs in Europe, funding existing research and development, as well as events and conferences, development of a quality plan, meetings for the exchange of best practices, virtual learning and networking, knowledge and recognition of European higher education credits ECTS (European Credit Transfer and Accumulation System).

The results of this project are on its website that we have indicated previously.

The COPOLAD Project for Latin America

The COPOLAD project is a cooperation program between the European Union and Latin America (www.copolad.eu) which began in 2011 and will last at least until 2025. It is intended to improve the coherence, balance, and impact of drug policies, through the exchange of experiences, bi-regional coordination, and the promotion of multisectoral, comprehensive, and coordinated responses. All with the idea of strengthening drug policies in Latin America (LA) and promoting cooperation between the national agencies responsible for policies in the countries of both regions.

It is financed by the EU and aims to: (1) consolidate the coordination and cooperation mechanisms on drugs between the EU and Latin America and the Caribbean through the bi-regional dialogue, (2) create or consolidate national drug observatories, (3) training for demand reduction, and (4) training for supply reduction. Its current areas of work are: drug observatory; problematic consumption; reduction of the illegal drug market; support for bi-regional coordination and cooperation on drugs; sustainable development, human rights, and gender; and innovation in drug policies.

The idea of this project is to facilitate dialogue, exchange of good practices, and training between the agencies in charge of formulating drug policies in Latin America and the European Union. To this end, they have developed a whole series of instruments, which can be consulted on their website, among which are the implementation of courses, preparation of documents, publication of manuals, exchange of technicians, holding systematic meetings for various topics, etc. This clearly favors the professional training of those responsible for developing and implementing the policies, of the professionals who have to put into practice the different prevention, treatment, and incorporation measures. The final objective is to reach consensus on evidence to achieve a series of quality standards for the planning, management, implementation, and evaluation of programs.

A good example of the above is the manual *Quality and evidence standards in drug demand reduction. Reference framework for program accreditation* (Salvador and Babín 2014). It contains the agreed criteria for prevention programs, for the reduction of risks associated with drug use, for treatment programs, for harm reduction programs, and for social incorporation programs. About 200 people participated in their preparation, from nine Latin American countries, along with Spain and Portugal and other international agencies from Europe and the United States. It is a good example of networking with tangible results. The rest of the materials have been made in the same line.

Publications and Research

The number of publications and research on prevention carried out in Europe is enormously extensive. Firstly, there are all the publications that the Lisbon European Monitoring Center for Drugs and Drug Addiction has. Everything it publishes is in electronic version. We indicate below some of the most relevant and recent ones, among the dozens that it has prepared (which can be downloaded at least in English from its website www.emcdda.europa.eu/publications):

- European drug report. Trends and news (2022)
- Hexahydrocannabinol (HHC) and related substances (2023)
- The future of drug monitoring in Europe until 2030 (2023)
- Women and drugs: health and social responses (2023)
- Families and drugs: health and social responses (2022)
- Homelessness and drugs: health and social responses (2022)
- Recreational use of nitrous oxide: A growing concern for Europe (2022)
- Prisons and drugs: health and social responses (2022)
- Schools and drugs: health and social responses (2022)
- Recreational settings and drugs: health and social responses (2022)
- Local communities and drugs: health and social responses (2022)
- Workplace and drugs: health and social responses (2022)

In addition, some previous publications stand out for the preventive field, such as those of:

- European drug prevention quality standards: A quick guide (2013)

- North American drug prevention programs: Are they feasible in European cultures and contexts? (2013)
- Guidelines for the evaluation of drug prevention: A manual for program planners and evaluators (second ed.) (2012)
- European drug prevention quality standards. Prevention profiles 2011 (2011)

At the same time, different countries, such as Spain, have a wide set of official publications, prepared by researchers, clinicians, or technicians, which they also have on their website. This is also favored because many of the projects and research financed by Spain's National Drug Plan, when published in book form, usually have an electronic version that can be accessed from the website of said National Plan. Below, we indicate those that we consider most important (all of which can be downloaded from www.pnsd.sanidad.gob.es):

- Family prevention of addictions. Challenges and opportunities of quality strategies (2022)
- European prevention curriculum. A handbook for decision-makers, opinion-makers and policy-makers on science-based prevention of substance use (2021)
- Guide to preventive strategies to reduce driving under the influence of alcohol and other psychoactive substances (2007)
- Scientific bases of drug addiction prevention (2002)
- Going out and drug use (2002)
- Family intervention in the prevention of drug addiction (2002)

From the "Acting is possible" collection of said organization, the manuals dedicated to how to act at school, family level, in the media, penitentiary centers, in primary health care, in social services, by the pharmacist, by forensic doctors, and in alcohol consumption. Also, within the Spanish Observatory on Drugs and Drug Addiction of the Spanish National Plan on Drugs, all epidemiology reports, drug indicators, drug supply and control, and international reports appear, which can be accessed through its website.

We also have different organizations, foundations, and European associations that are very active in preparing reports and studies related to the preventive field. Among the foundations that exist, we can take as an example the Mentor Foundation (http://mentorinternational.org/uk). In Europe it has several offices, such as in the United Kingdom, Germany, Sweden, and Lithuania; also in Latin American countries (e.g., Colombia), the Arabian Peninsula, and the United States. This foundation regularly collaborates with other European institutions and associations dedicated to drug prevention.

Conclusions and Projections

Europe is one of the continents with the highest drug consumption in the world, along with the United States of America. This increase has been developing in recent decades, similar to what has happened in other parts of the planet. When a problem arises it is necessary to address it. What has normally been done is to address the problem from the most visible part, which consists of providing treatment for the addict and making the supply of addictive substances difficult, leaving it until later to address the causes of the problem. But, to avoid the problems that drug use brings (treatment of dependency, associated physical illnesses, disorders mental problems, legal problems, social costs) this sanitary or repressive approach is not enough. It is necessary to put preventive measures into practice so that new cases do not appear or the appearance of associated problems is reduced as much as possible. However, in practice a lot of money is usually dedicated to the development of treatments for those affected, both sponsored by the administration and by pharmaceutical laboratories, or to repressive measures, and a preventive policy is delayed so that new cases do not appear. For those responsible, immediacy prevails, despite the fact that there are more and more studies that show the economic profitability of prevention compared to other more traditional measures. This occurs in almost all countries, although there are differences in the emphasis given to one orientation or another.

Despite what has been said, we know which measures are effective in preventing drug use, as summarized in Table 3, from the exhaustive review by Babor et al.

Table 3 Effective measures, based on scientific data, on what is effective in a drug policy

1. There is no single drug problem in the same society or in different societies; there is also no "magic formula" that will solve the drug problem
2. Many measures that influence drug problems are not considered drug policy and many specific drug policies have large effects outside the drug field
3. Activities promoted by developed countries to reduce the cultivation of drug-producing plants in poor countries have not decreased the global supply of drugs or their use in markets and probably never will
4. Once drugs have been made illegal, there is a point beyond which stricter law enforcement and incarceration produce very little additional benefit
5. Investments in proven services for opioid-dependent people generally reduce drug-related problems
6. School, family, and community prevention programs have modest effects
7. The drug policy debate is dominated in many countries by four false dichotomies that can confuse policymakers about the range of legitimate options and intended effects: (1) supposedly different methods of implementation of the law and health services (a distinction sometimes abbreviated to "police as opposed to doctors"; (2) policies that support services for drug users in contrast to those aimed at harm reduction; (3) the frequently drawn distinction between "good drugs" (legal and prescription drugs) and "bad drugs" (illegal drugs); and, (4) the presumed need for a reciprocal understanding between the interest of drug users and from the rest of society
8. The perverse effects of drug policy are common
9. The legal pharmaceutical system can influence the shape of a country's drug problem and the range of options available for drug policy
10. There is no scientific research that guides towards improving supply control and law enforcement activities

Source: Adapted from Babor et al. (2010)

(2010), or as other authors have indicated along the same lines (e.g., Strang et al. 2012). We are failing as prevention technicians or health professionals, in the social field or in the educational field, to convince public officials to dedicate more money, efforts, and attention to the prevention of drug use. This clashes with the interests of the tobacco and alcohol industry, and other industries such as leisure and free time, or restaurants, which do not want control over people's access to behaviors that may be excessive or problematic (such as excessive alcohol consumption). We are also assisting the important interests of the cannabis industry, which is effectively influencing public opinion and the political agenda.

We have enough scientific information to know what needs to be done, about effective programs, what actions are not desirable, how to implement them in the most efficient way, etc. In practice this is not always done. For this reason, we need to share the work between different countries, professionals, applicators of programs, and evaluators, in order to ensure that this field gains the relevance it deserves, to prevent many people from having serious health problems, physical and mental, due to the consumption of drugs.

In Europe, much progress has been made in the field of drugs, in terms of prevention and treatment, although in recent years there has been stagnation or regression in the preventive field in some countries. This has been happening because the treatment has gained enormous relevance in a short time, with the appearance of different drugs—often with very dubious efficacy in terms of addictions—and with the interested promotion of pharmaceutical laboratories and certain biological psychiatric sectors with what they call "dual pathology" (in many cases the dual pathology is the result of consumption, disappearing when it is stopped), converting almost all addicts into a "mentally ill" person due to the associated comorbidity that they frequently have. But not all users are addicts. And, the preventive field suffers if what is transmitted is that we are facing a "disease," not a behavior that can be avoided and, above all, that can be effectively prevented. At the same time, the money dedicated to prevention has decreased in different countries due to the economic crisis that has been experienced in many European countries since 2007, and more currently due to the Covid-19 epidemic, and the invasion of Ukraine by Russia.

Critical and interested voices have also emerged about the effectiveness of prevention. It is a good attack system when you want to sink something specific, discredit, or create doubts. These criticisms have arisen from some sectors of biological treatment, and from other sectors of consumers and associations active in harm reduction or pro-legalization of drug consumption, especially cannabis. This creates a breeding ground where confusion can lead to doubt and nothing could be decided. Luckily, we have effective preventive programs, competent technicians, and adequate preventive technology. But this is not always put into practice, it is not always applied at the necessary level of intensity, or different types of restrictions are put in place.

But the truth is that a society cannot give up prevention (National Academies of Sciences, Engineering, and Medicine [NASEM] 2019). Prevention is part of any human social system. Our forecast for the future of prevention in Europe is specified in the following aspects:

- The alcohol industry tries to get involved in prevention. But what they are doing is counter-prevention. An example of this is the Spanish spirits federation, FEBE (www.febe.es), which offers its preventive program free of charge to public and private institutions and to anyone who wants to implement it, and free of charge through the Alcohol and Society Foundation. In other countries, their alternative or designated driver campaigns stand out (a sober driver, even if he has the others in the car who are drunk). Practices that we believed to be in the past are now being put into practice again, sponsored by the alcohol industry, due to the economic crisis and public administrations investing less money in prevention.
- We must also take into account the very powerful nightlife industry, whose interests also go hand in hand in many issues with the city councils and regional governments themselves also eager to attract young people and increase their tax earnings.
- There is an important pro-legalization movement of cannabis in several European countries, as in other places in the world, which facilitates or opens the door to the legalization of so-called recreational cannabis. This confuses, or attempts to hide from the population, the negative and sometimes serious consequences of cannabis use—especially among adolescents—such as its high prevalence and increase in treatment demands. The issue is raised as if consumption were normal. The clear economic interests that underlie its liberalization or use for recreational purposes, the demagoguery of tax collection, are hidden, and an interested confusion arises about the supposed therapeutic properties (Volkow et al. 2014). All of this encourages a debate that has been growing in recent years and will continue to be maintained.
- It is important to know the risk and protective factors for drug consumption, in each specific context, in each country, in each region, in each city. Knowing them is of great importance for the application of preventive programs and also for the development of new preventive programs.
- Progress will continue in knowing what are the essential elements that a good preventive program must have. Although we know the most relevant ones (Becoña 2002), the future advancement of the field of prevention is along these lines because we need to know and act on the central ones. This will result in being able to develop better preventive programs and, therefore, make them more effective.
- Related to all of the above, the need for what we know as "evidence-based prevention"or "good prevention practices" is increasingly assumed. In the coming years this will become even more relevant in different European countries. Knowing what works, under what conditions it works, and for whom it works is central to our field (Faggiano et al. 2014; MacArthur et al. 2018).

- Environmental prevention is a central element within the preventive field (Burkhart 2011). Its implementation is very effective, and makes it easier to put into practice other types of prevention (Becoña 2021). But for it to be implemented, a social culture of prevention is needed, which is lacking in many countries.
- It is necessary to transmit more intensely to the entire hedonistic society in which we live the negative consequences of drug consumption (Calafat 2010). When the recreational life model was implemented in young people and some adults in many European countries, which is linked to the consumption of alcohol and drugs, it has led to the negative consequences of drug consumption skyrocketing in recent decades. This new way of consuming, closely linked to weekend recreational contexts, opens the door for many "normalized" young people with a good social fabric to consume. The feeling of problems—violence, unwanted sexual relations, traffic accidents—linked to these consumptions disappears easily (Calafat et al. 2000, 2008a). To reverse this situation, information, awareness, and social norms are needed to counteract these consequences. It is a long task for professionals of prevention.
- It is necessary to achieve greater coordination and European integration on the issue of drug prevention. Much progress has been made and it is to be hoped that this harmonization will continue in the coming years. Steps have been taken and will continue to be done in the coming years.

References

Becoña, E. (1999). *Bases teóricas que sustentan los programas de prevención de drogas*. Madrid: Delegación del Gobierno para el Plan Nacional sobre Drogas, Ministerio del Interior.

Becoña, E. (2002). *Bases científicas de la prevención de las drogodependencias*. Madrid: Delegación del Gobierno para el Plan Nacional sobre Drogas, Ministerio del Interior.

Becoña, E. (2021). *La Prevención Ambiental en el Consumo de Drogas. ¿Qué medidas podemos aplicar?* Madrid: Ministerio de Sanidad. Delegación del Gobierno para el Plan Nacional sobre Drogas-

Babor, T., Caulkins, J., Edwards, G., Fischer, B., Foxcroft, D., Huamphreys, K. et al. (2010). *La política de drogas y el bien público*. Washington, DC: Organización Panamericana de Salud.

Burkhart, G. (2011). Prevención ambiental de drogas en la Unión Europea. ¿Por qué es tan impopular este tipo de prevención? *Adicciones, 23*, 87-100.

Calafat, A. (2010). *Prevention interventions in recreational settings*. Strasbourg: Council of Europe. Pompidou Group.

Calafat, A.; Amengual, M.; Mejias, G.; Borras, M. y Palmer, A. (1989). Evaluación del programa de prevención escolar 'Tú decides'". *Adicciones. 1*, 96-111.

Calafat, A., Amengual, M. y Farrés, C. (1985). *Tú decides. Manual del profesor*. Palma de Mallorca: Conseil Insular.

Calafat, A., Amengual, M., Farrés, C. y Borrás, M. (2008a) *Tú decides*. Palma de Mallorca: Conseil Insular.

Calafat, A., Becoña, E., Duch, M. y Juan, M. (2023). *Tú decides. 2.0*. Palma de Mallorca: IREFREA.

Calafat, A., Duch, M., Juan, M. y Leckenby, N. (2012). Health and safety European standards for nightlife venues. *Adicciones, 24*, 355-364.

Calafat, A., Fernández, C., Juan, M., y Becoña, E. (2008b) Recreational nightlife: Risk and protective factors for drug misuse among young Europeans in recreational environments. *Drugs: education, prevention and policy 15 (2)*, 189-200.

Calafat, A., Juan, M., Becoña, E., Fernández, C., Gil, E., Palmer, A., Sureda, P., & Torres, M.A. (2000) *Salir de marcha y consumo de drogas*. Madrid, Plan Nacional sobre Drogas.

Caria, M. P., Faggiano, F., Bellocco, R., & Galanti, M. R. (2011a). The influence of socioeconomic environment on the effectiveness of alcohol prevention among European students: A cluster randomized controlled trial. *BMC Public Health, 11*, 312. doi https://doi.org/10.1186/1471-2458-11-312

Caria, M. P., Faggiano, F., Bellocco, R., Galanti, M. R., & EU-Dap Study Group (2011b). Effects of a school-based prevention program on European adolescents' patterns of alcohol use. *Journal of Adolescent Health, 48,* 182-188.

Culley, D. M., Taylor, J., Rubin, J., Hoorens, S., Disley, E., & Rabinovich, L. (2012). *Assessment of the implementation of the EU drugs strategy 2005-2012 and its action plans*. Santa Monica, CA: Rand Corporation.

ESPAD Group (2020). *ESPAD Report 2019: Results from the European School Survey Project on Alcohol and Other Drugs*. EMCDDA Joint Publications Office of the European Union, Luxembourg.

European Commission. Directorate General for Justice (2022). Impact of drugs on communitie. In: https://europa.eu/eurobarometer/surveys/detail/2281

European Monitoring Centre for Drugs and Drug Addiction [EMCDDA] (2011). *European drug prevention quality standards. A manual for prevention professionals*. Lisboa: European Monitoring Centre for Drugs and Drug Addiction.

Faggiano, F., Galanti, M. R., Bohrn, M. R., Burkhart, G., Vigna-Taglianti, F., Cuomo, L., …EU-Dap Study Group (2008). The effectiveness of a school-based substance abuse prevention program: EU-Dap cluster randomized controlled trial. *Preventive Medicine, 47*, 537-543.

Faggiano, F., Allara, E. Giannotta, F., Molinar, R., Summall H., Wiers, R.,... Conrod, P. (2014). Europe needs a central, transparent, and evidence-based approval process for behavioural prevention interventions. *Plos Medicine, 11,* 21001740.

Ferri, M., & Bo, A. (2013). Best practice promotion in Europe: A web-based tool for the dissemination of evidence-based demand reduction interventions. *Drugs: Education, Prevention and Policy, 20,* 331-337.

Frances, A. (2014). *¿Somos todos enfermos mentales?* Madrid: Ariel.

Giannotta, F., Vigna-Taglianti, F., Galanti, M. R., Scatigna, M., & Faggiano, F. (2014). Short-term mediating factors of a school-based intervention to prevent youth substance use in Europe. *Journal of Adolescent Health, 54*, 565-573. doi https://doi.org/10.1016/j.jadohealth.2013.10.009

Gotzsche, P. C. (2014). *Medicamentos que matan y crimen organizado. Cómo las grandes farmacéuticas han corrompido el sistema de salud.* Barcelona: Los libros del lince.

Juan, M., Calafat, A., Duch, M., & Guerrero, M. A. (2018). *Programa Ferya. Familias en red y activas. Programa de empoderamiento familiar para prevenir los riesgos que afectan a los menores*. Palma de Mallorca. Irefrea.

Kornblit, A. L., Mendes, A. M., & Bilyk, A. (1990). "'Vos decidis': un programa de prevención de consumo de drogas en la escuela media". *Medicina y Sociedad, 13 (5-6)*, 36-40.

Macià, D., Olivares, J., & Méndez, F. X. (1993). Intervención comportamental-educativa en la prevención de la drogodependencia. In F. X. Méndez, D. Maciá, D. y J. Olivares. *Intervención conductual en contextos comunitarios I. Programas aplicados de prevención*. Madrid: Pirámide.

Mackenbach, J. P., & McKee, M. (2013). A comparative analysis of health policy performance in 43 European countries. *European Journal of Public Health, 23,* 195–344. doi:https://doi.org/10.1093/eurpub/cks192).

MacArthur, G., Caldwell, D. M., Redmore, J., Watkins, S. H., Kipping, R., White, J., ..., Campbell, R. (2018). Individual-, family-, and school-level intervention targeting multiple risk behaviours in young people. *Cochrane Dababase of Systematic Review, Issue 10*, Art. No. CD009927.

National Academies of Sciences, Engineering, and Medicine [NASEM] (2019). *Fostering healthy mental, emotional, and behavioral development in children and youth: A national agenda.* Washington, DC: The National Academies Press.

O'Connell, M. E., Boat, T., & Warner, K. E. (Eds.) (2009). *Preventing mental, emotional and behavioral disorders among young people. Progress and possibilities.* Washington, DC: National Academies Press

Oncioiu, S. I., Burkhart, G., Calafat, A., Duch, M., Perman-Howe, P., & Foxcroft, D. R. (2018). *Environmental substance use prevention interventions in Europe.* Lisboa: EMCDDA.

Rödner, S., Olsson, B., & Room, R. (Eds.) (2008). *A cannabis reader: Global issues and local experiences, vol. 1.* Lisboa: European Monitoring Centre for Drugs and Drug Addiction.

Rodríguez-Martos, A., Torralba, LL., & Vecino, C. (1996). Decideix! Programa de prevención del abuso de drogas en enseñanza secundaria: la experiencia de Barcelona. *Adicciones, 8*, 127-148.

Salvador, T., & Babín, F. (2014). *Calidad y evidencia en reducción de la demanda de drogas. Marco de referencia para la acreditación de programas.* Madrid: COPOLAD.

Strang, J., Babor, T., Caulkins, J., Fischer, B., Foxcroft, D., & Humphreys, K. (2012). Drug policy and the public good: Evidence for effective interventions. *Lancet, 379*, 71-83.

United Nations (2007). *Sweden's successful drug policy: A review of the evidence.* New York NY: United Nations, Office on Drug and Crime.

UNODOC (2013). *International standards on drug use prevention.* New York: United Nations on Drugs and Crime.

UNODOC (2018). *International standards on drug use prevention, 2nd ed. updated.* New York: United Nations on Drugs and Crime.

Vadrucci, S., Vigna-Taglianti, F. D., van der Kreeft, P., Vassara, M., Scatigna, M., Faggiano, F., Burkhart, G., & EU-Dap Study Group (2016). The theoretical model of the school-based prevention programme Unplugged. *Global Health Promotion, 23(4),* 49–58.

Van der Kreeft, P., Wiborg, G., Galanti, M. R., Siliquini, R., Bohrn, K., Castigna, M., ... EU-Dap Study Group (2009). "Unplugged": A new European school programme against substance abuse. *Drug: Education, Prevention and Policy, 16,* 167-181.

Vigna-Taglianti, F. D., Galanti, M. R., Burkhart, G., Caria, M. P., Vadrucci, S. Faggiano, F....for the EU-Dap Study Group (2014). "Unplugged", a European school-based program for substance use prevention among adolescents: Overview of results from the EU-Dap trial. In G. G. Noam, K. Weichold y F. Giannotta (Eds.), *Theory-based approaches to substance misuse and abuse prevention in school* (pp. 67-82). San Francisco, CA: Jossey-Bass.

Villalbí, J. R., Bosque-Prous, M., Gili-Miner, M., Espelt, A., & Brugal, M. T. (2014). Políticas para prevenir los daños causados por el alcohol. *Revista Española de Salud Pública, 88,* 515-528.

Volkow, N. D., Baler, R. D., Compton, W. M., & Weiss, S. R. B. (2014). Adverse health effects of marijuana use. *New England Journal of Medicine, 370*, 2219-2227.

Evidence-Based Prevention: Effective Approaches for Drug Demand Reduction in Mexico

José Luis Benítez Villa and Carmen Fernández Cáceres

Country Context

Mexico is a country located in North America that shares borders with the United States to the north, and Guatemala and Belize to the southeast. It has a territorial area that covers approximately 1,964,375km^2 and a population of more than 120 million inhabitants, making it the most populous Spanish-speaking country in the world. Mexico is home to a rich ethnic and cultural diversity, with a mix of indigenous, European and African heritage. In addition, it has great biodiversity, with tropical jungles, deserts, mangroves, and rich marine life on its coasts bathed by two oceans. With a diversified economy that includes agriculture, manufacturing, and tourism, Mexico is a regional power with an important role in global politics and the economy.

Introduction

Evidence-based practice, a paradigm rooted in the search and application of solid and verifiable data, which has its roots in so-called evidence-based medicine, has revolutionized the way knowledge and decision-making are approached in various areas. Originally, during the second half of the twentieth century, this perspective arose in response to the need for a more rigorous method to adopt clinical determinations, by establishing a reliable link between medical interventions and the real results in the health of patients (Guyatt et al. 1992). However, its evolution has been

J. L. B. Villa (✉) · C. F. Cáceres
Centros de Integración Juvenil (CIJ), Mexico City, Mexico
e-mail: jose.benitez@cij.gob.mx; cfernandez@cij.gob.mx

A. Pérez-Gómez, J. Mejía-Trujillo (eds.), *Drug Abuse Prevention*, Advances in Mental Health and Addiction, https://doi.org/10.1007/978-3-031-99621-4_5

guided by advances in research and the growing availability of data through new technologies, until it has become a methodology to support decisions and actions in public health based on objective and reliable information; challenging traditional practices based on intuition and individual experience that do not have scientific support (Jenicek 1997; Lhachimi et al. 2016).

The acceptance and robustness of the evidence-based approach has not only established a milestone in the medical field, but has expanded to various disciplines. Among other areas of knowledge, it is used in psychology to support therapeutic approaches; in education, it bases the implementation of effective pedagogical models; in sociology, it helps understand social patterns more accurately; in economics, it allows formulating policies based on data; and in scientific research in general, it has become a guiding principle to face challenges and guarantee the validity of the findings (Hoffmann and Glasziou 2016).

The range of possible transdisciplinary applications of evidence-based practice is broad. However, its essential philosophy is shared: It lies in the constant and systematic search for the best available information, critical analysis of data before any election, and the adaptation of actions based on specific results (Smith and Rennie 2014). The above establishes a bridge between theory and effective practice, in a variety of contexts that, in physical and mental health care, encompasses the treatment of existing diseases and conditions, as well as a fundamental preventive dimension for sustainable well-being; including the mitigation of risk factors, active health promotion, adoption of healthy lifestyles, and reduction of preventable diseases.

Evolution of Approaches to Addiction Care

The prevalence and trends of drug consumption, reported through global reports, national surveys, and data from epidemiological surveillance systems, show variations over the years that reflect that the supply and demand of psychoactive substances are part of a phenomenon dynamic in constant transformation (United Nations Office on Drugs and Crime [UNODC] 2023; Youth Integration Centers [CIJ] 2023; INPRFM et al. 2017a, b, c). The studies show how consumption patterns change over time, in different geographical environments and contextual frameworks; they offer information on the magnitude of the problem, types of psychoactive substances used, and emerging challenges that require attention, but they also reveal how cultural and economic factors and aspects linked to the regulation of psychoactive substances shape behaviors related to them. Ultimately, interpreting the data from the reports captures the current landscape and current actions, while guiding decision making toward a healthier future. In this way, the knowledge resulting from these works is a source to identify and develop therapeutic approaches, as well as establish a link with the prevention of addictions, since, from a population perspective, the epidemiological profiles are consistent and potentially predictable;

this makes it possible to identify opportunities for intervention and anticipate adverse outcomes (Griffin and Botvin 2010).

According to data from the National Survey on Drug, Alcohol, and Tobacco Consumption (ENCODAT) 2016–2017, carried out in Mexico, the prevalence of use of psychoactive substances progressively increases during adolescence, reaching its peak in the first years of adult life and decreases in subsequent years. Also, it is proven that the onset of substance use at an early age contributes to higher levels of use and abuse in adulthood (INPRFM et al. 2017a, b, c). Likewise, it is associated with negative behavioral, social, and health outcomes, including physical and mental health problems; aggressive and violent behaviors; and adaptation difficulties in the family, work, and community environment, throughout their life (Degenhardt et al. 2018). Thus, by understanding the characteristics of consumption, the progression to drug use disorders, and the underlying factors, it is possible to develop preventive strategies in a precise and strategic manner, focusing on the most susceptible contexts and populations, as well as on the moments and delivery devices most suitable for implementation (Newcomb and Locke 2005).

Nowadays, there is consensus in the scientific community and in the academic field that the most efficient and effective strategies to prevent the consumption of psychoactive substances are those focused on modifying risk factors and promoting protective ones, at the individual, family, and/or community level; while they must be guided by relevant psychosocial theories on the etiology of drug use and abuse (Substance Abuse and Mental Health Services Administration [SAMHSA] 2019). Hence, the objectives of the programs range from preventing or delaying behaviors related to consumption; limit the number of substances used; avoid the transition from experimenting with substance use to abuse and dependence; reduce the negative consequences in those who have already used them or who progress to disorders due to their use; educate people so that they are able to maintain a mature and responsible relationship with drugs; stimulate the psychosocial development and well-being of individuals throughout their lives; and modify the conditions of the sociocultural environment to promote healthy development alternatives (Fernández et al. 2022). However, having solid theoretical bases and integrating this evidence has required the evolution of explanatory models of the phenomenon of addictions. The changes in this conceptualization have set the tone to generate, test, modify, enrich, and improve the guidelines of preventive programs that have emerged over the years in different latitudes of the world, including Mexico; some of which continue to operate. Therefore, it is essential to understand the bases of these approaches, since they were decisive for the formation of contemporary preventive approaches.

Legal Ethical Model

In the sixties, the predominant theoretical model aimed at understanding the "problem" of drug use was the ethical-legal one, based on the belief that addictions have moral and behavioral roots. In this case, the substance is assigned the role of causal agent and, therefore, a predominant place in the configuration of the problem. For their part, the person is placed in the background, and judgments are prescribed that arise from an assessment of what is good, what is bad, what is permitted, and what is prohibited. In this case, it is considered that drug users are responsible for their actions and addictive behavior must be punished, in defense of social order; he is therefore a transgressor, a criminal who is stigmatized and punished (Ministry of Education of the Nation 2009).

The preventive discourse that results from this approach emphasizes that the use of psychoactive drugs is illegal and morally unacceptable, defending their prohibition and abstinence. Therefore, preventive actions are aimed at reducing supply, compliance with the laws, combating and punishing drug trafficking; supervision of production and distribution; determination of penalties for participating in the production, sale, and consumption of substances and the establishment of conventions and agreements to combat all aspects of this phenomenon. From this perspective, the belief is assumed that the population does not know the effects of consumption, but that, if sensitized on the subject, they would be able to make the decision to avoid it (Becoña 1999). For this reason, information is used so that individuals know the legal and moral consequences and penalties of the use and distribution of psychoactive substances. In this approach, the concept of authority that legislates and sanctions is reinforced. Prevention is assimilated to control; the warning, fear, and moralistic content being the elements that seek to discourage consumption.

With respect to this perspective, among its deficiencies is that the transmission of information may be inappropriate for certain ages or generate confusion, increasing the curiosity of the population at risk, and without affecting those who already have a history of drug use. However, the ethical-legal model can play an important role in preventing addictions in certain contexts. Regulations and legal restrictions on the advertising and sale of controlled substances, for example, can help reduce the availability and access to certain drugs, especially among younger people.

Medical-Health Model

During the seventies, the medical-care approach emerged, a significant milestone in the understanding of addictions, both for its prevention and its treatment. This vision migrates from a moral perception to one of a scientific nature, oriented towards health, which was developed in parallel with the advances in research on the effects of psychoactive drugs on the brain and nervous system. The above raised the hypothesis that addictions have a biological basis, so they should be considered diseases with their own course and different stages (natural history); where changes in the brain play a crucial role in drug-associated compulsion and loss of control (Uhl et al. 2019). Like the previous model, the emphasis is placed on the substance, but understood as an agent that induces the disease in the presence of a state of individual susceptibility, which is inserted in an environment that favors consumption. The drug user is no longer seen as a criminal, but as sick: They are a person who was healthy and who became ill due to substance use. The identification of the agent will no longer occur based on normative-moral criteria, but rather based on its toxicity or addictive potential, which supports the reduction of stigma about people who use drugs.

One of the key moments in the emergence of the healthcare approach was the classification of addictions as a disease, in the Diagnostic and Statistical Manual of Mental Disorders (Robinson and Adinoff 2016; American Psychiatric Association 1994). Thus, the idea was legitimized that, since it is a health issue, it requires clinical attention; bringing with it the development of pharmacological treatments to reduce withdrawal symptoms and the intense desire to consume substances. Also, it influenced prevention, by emphasizing the importance of education about the harms caused by drug use, highlighting the short-term harms. The interventions are based on the reinforcement of values, self-esteem, beliefs, and attitudes. It seeks to change the positive conception and expectations about substance use, with a negative vision. Therefore, it becomes common to transmit messages with exhaustive descriptions of the appearance, forms of presentation, routes of consumption, and effects of drugs on the body (chronic, irreversible, disabling, lethal disorders). It is recommended that people recognize the substances and identify the profile and presence of a consumer (Tavera and Martínez s/f). By virtue of the above, the typical preventive activity of this model is the discussion or conference, chaired, in general, by a doctor who clearly marks his place as a specialist and role as an expert, in a vertical relationship with a public that "does not know" about the topic. Furthermore, this theoretical perspective promotes the idea that addictions should be addressed as a public health issue, which led to the creation of programs and policies aimed at the prevention, treatment, and rehabilitation of drug users. In summary, the emergence of the medical-care model marked a fundamental change in the perception of addictions, by recognizing its biological basis and promoting medical and therapeutic care as essential components for effective prevention and treatment.

Even considering the contributions of the medical-care vision, limitations have also been attributed to it. It has been pointed out that one of the "dangers" of this perspective is that the toxic effects of drugs can be overstated, which, when trying to dissuade through fear, can result in the loss of credibility of the messages, making communication difficult. When faced with a sender who "lies," the receiver could choose "not to listen" (Ministry of Education of the Nation 2009). Furthermore, it must be taken into account that the components of the addiction phenomenon are not completely understood from a medical perspective. Multidisciplinary models that consider psychosocial and contextual factors are essential for effective prevention and sustainable recovery. Likewise, this approach can neglect cultural and social aspects that influence the appearance and development of substance use disorders.

Sociocultural Model

As research and experience revealed the complexity of addictions, it became evident that these disorders cannot be addressed solely from an individual or medical perspective, which led to the adoption of alternative models in the 1980s, such as sociocultural models. In this case, we seek to explain drug use from the social and cultural organization that, with economic structures and circumstantial aspects, determine collective processes. According to this criterion, addictions are an expression of individuals' discomfort when faced with environments or events that do not cover their basic needs. Thus, factors such as peer influence, availability of substances, stress, economic vulnerability, overcrowding, marginalization, urbanization, industrialization, unemployment, cultural movements, and social norms play an outstanding role in the initiation and development of addictions. That is, for the sociocultural model, the context is the problem axis and, therefore, the reading is carried out from a macrosocial or socio-community dimension that refers to the broader social and institutional environment and is related to the economic structure legal and normative of a society, or with the socio-community dynamics. According to this approach, it is in the social environment where the causes of drug consumption must be sought. In response to the adoption of the sociocultural perspective, prevention strategies focus on changing the environment to reduce risk factors and strengthen protective factors; promoting a holistic approach that treats addictive behavior, its social and cultural roots. Therefore, a preventive project built from this approach requires intervention in state policies, to promote the development of the community; that is, carrying out activities that improve housing conditions, public service infrastructure, access to health, education, culture, and employment opportunities, as well as changes in social structures and relationships.

Now, it is unavoidable that when adopting this perspective and considering the approach of addressing addictions in a particular context, a detailed understanding of the environment where the population lives to which the efforts will be directed is required, so the identification of its characteristics, through research, becomes a necessary requirement. In Mexico, studies have been carried out that have investigated sociodemographic variables, education, migration, crime, and violence (Nevárez Sida et al. 2022; Sánchez Hoil et al. 2017; Arellanez 2016; Díaz Negrete and García Aurrecoechea 2008). These investigations contribute to the understanding of the socio-community challenges that the country faces in relation to drugs, highlighting the urgency of addressing not only consumption, but also the network of social and economic aspects in a comprehensive manner. Likewise, there are documented studies that have evaluated macrosocial risks related to the use of psychoactive drugs, at the level of the states and municipalities of the Mexican Republic. These analyses provide evidence on the complex dynamics of this phenomenon, by identifying a wide range of presentations and factors involved in the same problem, in a single country, but with differences when examined in local contexts (Rodríguez-Kuri et al. 2019; García Aurrecoechea et al. 2016; Salinas et al. 1997).

Also, the so-called Basic Objective Community Study (EBCO) is a diagnostic source on drug consumption, sociodemographic conditions, and the social response organized in specific geographical locations (CIJ 2019). Its objective is to support the planning, formulation, and application of lines of action, programs, and addiction care services in areas of influence, at specific times. This is how data has resulted in the rational administration of resources intended to address addictions, by supporting decision-making to implement preventive actions at strategic points that reach more people, as well as the creation of therapeutic care units for places in greater vulnerability.

On the other hand, it is worth noting that, in the evolution of preventive models, until before this decade, the strategies proposed the approach in a broad sense, without a precise focus on the underlying causes or on the population groups at greatest risk. This generic conception did not have the capacity to identify and effectively treat particular threats to health, which led to dividing substance use prevention programs, adapting the proposal on the natural history of the disease, into levels traditionally categorized as primary, secondary, and tertiary (Sánchez and Velasco 2017). Primary prevention acts in the prepathogenic period and is aimed at preventing the problem from arising; specifically, it focuses on preventing the population from engaging in drug use in the first place. For its part, secondary prevention focuses on early identification, attention, and minimizing consequences when consumption has been experienced and the problem manifests itself. Finally, tertiary prevention is aimed at treating and rehabilitating people who progress to substance use disorders. This differentiation arose with the intention of precisely and strategically planning the programs, leading to more effective results in the promotion and maintenance of health throughout life (Becoña 2002). However, this classification has been the subject of debate and criticism, among other reasons, because it is considered that it was developed under a strictly medical vision; for running the risk of oversimplifying the complexity of addictions, the lack of focus on early intervention; and given the need for adaptation in specific contexts. Thus, new knowledge and practices evolved over time towards a more comprehensive and evidence-based perspective that recognizes the interaction of biological, psychological, social, and environmental factors in the development and perpetuation of addiction (Moscoso and Titto 2015; Hopenhayn 2002).

Psychosocial Model

In parallel to the sociocultural approach, the psychosocial perspective emerged in the 1990s as a fundamental pillar in understanding and addressing this health challenge. This approach does not place emphasis on drugs, but on people, who define their behavioral repertoire based on the presence or absence of factors that increase or decrease the statistical probability of developing disorders associated with substance use. From this perspective, the identification of risk and protective factors (of a biological, psychological, environmental, and social nature, which reside at the individual, family, community, and institutional level) is extremely useful to act on these variables. In such a way that risk and protection factors are not opposite entities on a continuum, but rather two differentiated realities that interact with each other (Nawi et al. 2021).

In the psychosocial vision, the axis of the cause of the problem is changed: Addiction is not the disease, but the manifestation of a psychological disorder. The individual becomes the protagonist and the link established with the drug is highlighted, with what are considered concepts of use, abuse, and dependence, as well as patterns limited to the frequency of substance consumption, regardless of their legal or pharmacological status. The psychosocial approach, therefore, conceives addictions as behavioral disorders that arise as a mechanism to resolve conflicts of the person in their microsocial environment, for which they do not have sufficient individual and social tools to deal with them. In this way, it considers membership and reference groups as essential agents that can influence the development and prevention of addictions, with special emphasis on the family, school, and peer group. Consequently, the strategies do not recognize the exclusive purpose of avoiding drug use; they go beyond rejecting consumption; its objectives focus on the emotional development and general and specific skills (Becoña 1999). In this scenario, measures that strengthen resilience are emphasized, so that people are able to handle adverse situations. The above, through psychoeducational interventions, are based on sociocognitive models, social relearning methods, and behavioral modeling techniques that focus their actions on self-care, improvement of interpersonal relationships, promotion of healthy lifestyles, activities for comprehensive health and human and personal development.

In this decade, life skills programs stand out, aimed at strengthening the skills necessary to effectively face the challenges of daily life, through social or interpersonal skills, including communication, negotiation/rejection strategies, trust, cooperation, and empathy; cognitive skills, such as problem solving, understanding consequences, decision making, critical thinking, and self-evaluation; and healthy emotion management, namely, stress management and self-monitoring (Mangrulkar et al. 2001). Also, programs with an educational focus that reinforce competencies stand out, such as the Positive Development of Adolescents, which highlights positive resources and potential, instead of focusing on combating the supposed disabilities of young people (CIJ 2015). Thus, we work on prosocial behaviors and the skills necessary to be successful in the school, work, and community settings; avoid or delay the onset of substance use, prevent risky sexual practices, promote positive social adjustment; as well as identifying and managing emotions in a healthy way. Likewise, the model of social and emotional competencies becomes relevant, which outlines the characteristics necessary for young people to become successful adults (Lerner 2005).

In the timeline, in this period prevention stops focusing solely on the issue of drugs and joins a much more robust framework: the field of mental health. Furthermore, given the limitations of the model, which classified actions into primary, secondary, and tertiary prevention levels, the National Research Council and Institute of Medicine of the United States of America formulated a new framework for the prevention of the use of psychoactive drugs based on in the contributions made by different authors within the field of mental health prevention (Newhouse and Spring 2010; Leaf 1999). In this proposal, the types of prevention are configured according to the population they are aimed at. Then, based on the risk and protective factors approach, interventions are classified as universal, selective, and indicated. Universal prevention is aimed at the general population, without distinguishing their level of risk for drug use; implements global strategies to promote healthy practices and avoid consumption; it has low cost, wide coverage, and does not require specialized training for its operation. Selective prevention is aimed at groups exposed to psychosocial conditions associated with consumption. Risk factors can be biological, psychological, social, or environmental; the objective is to delay the first contact with the drug and the age at which its use begins. The actions and content are delimited based on the elements that are a threat to this population and requires specialized personnel. On the other hand, the indicated prevention is aimed at those who have experimented with psychoactive substances, show associated problematic behaviors or are exposed to situations of psychosocial risk, but who do not meet the criteria of abuse or dependence. The objectives are focused on preventing the transition from experimentation or occasional use to addiction and reducing the effects and consequences that consumption could generate (Fernández et al. 2022; Harrop and Catalano 2016). This conceptual precision allows us to propose care strategies in accordance with the levels and types of risk of each population, in different social settings. Table 1 presents some pioneering research from Mexico that explored the role of psychosocial risk factors associated with drug use.

Ecological/Integrative Model

The evolution of the concept of health until its conception as a state that encompasses aspects of physical and mental well-being, ability to function, adaptation, and active participation in the social life of the community where a person lives, was accompanied by the development of explanatory models on the elements that affect maintaining health, preventing disease, or restoring the state of balance. Thus, from an integrative intention, interest in ecological approaches is consolidated, a proposal that, rather than attempting to establish causal relationships, takes into account different levels of interaction between the person and their environment, namely: (a) the environment, in relation to the natural environment and especially the social context; (b) the styles and habits of life, where the behaviors and habits that are formed by personal decisions and by influences of the environment and social group are considered and that in a given moment, they can negatively affect health; (c) the health system, subject to variables such as accessibility, efficiency and effectiveness, centers and resources, as well as good practices and coverage; and (d) human biology, which includes genetic load and hereditary factors (De La Guardia Gutiérrez and Ruvalcaba Ledezma 2020).

Table 1 Research on psychosocial factors associated with drug consumption in Mexico

Authors	Identified psychosocial factors
Castro (1990)	Access to drugs or places where they are available; substance use in the peer group; favorable attitude to consumption; availability of money for personal use; school tolerance of drug use, lack of full-time dedication to studies; low parental support and control, substance use in the family, chaotic or disorganized family relationships; being a man; antisocial behavior; dissatisfaction with quality of life; nonconformity; traumatic or negative events from childhood and/or adolescence
Nazar et al. (1994)	Have friends who use drugs; father's drug use
Rodríguez et al. (1998)	Impulsiveness and aggressiveness; affective disorders and other psychological symptoms; connection with drug-using friends; antisocial attitudes and behaviors; low school adherence; inappropriate use of free time
Castro and Llanes (2001)	Emigration from rural to urban areas; work on the street; access to drugs or places where they are available; drug use in the peer group; favorable attitude to consumption; availability of money to buy drugs; school tolerance of substance use, lack of full-time dedication to studies, school problems in second childhood, loss of sense of belonging at school; weak family support and control, drug use in the family, chaotic or disorganized family, lack of contact with the family, parental divorce, loss of sense of belonging in the family; antisocial acts; dissatisfaction with quality of life; nonconformity; traumatic or negative childhood or recent events; close losses; suicidal ideation and attempts; early start of sexual life, early pregnancy, abortion, neglect of health and sexual life
Medina-Mora et al. (2003)	Not study; consider it easy to get drugs; tolerance of consumption by friends; substance use in the family and peer group; depression
Villatoro et al. (2004)	Low risk perception; do not dedicate full time to studying
Arellanez et al. (2004)	Separation and breakdown of the family nucleus, dysfunctional family communication, family distancing; school adjustment problems; poor coping strategies; depressive symptoms, suicidal ideation and attempts; perceived accessibility to substances and low perceived risk of drug use
Rodríguez et al. (2007)	Favorable attitude and expectations regarding drug use; low perceived behavioral control in situations that favor the use of psychoactive substances
Díaz et al. (2009)	Depression; maladaptive school adjustment; maladaptive family cohesion and flexibility, high perceived impact of stress caused by family separation, dysfunctional family communication
Córdova et al. (2010)	Unsatisfactory perception of the quality of life (in particular, the use of free time and economic Well-being); difficulties with interaction; low self-esteem, depressed mood and negative affects; lack of hope and life project
Pérez and Díaz (2011)	Greater impact of perceived social violence and insecurity, less self-care, greater severity of anxiety and depression symptoms

In this context, the paradigm of the "Social Determinants of Health" gains popularity, defined as the circumstances in which people are born, grow, live, work, and age, which are the result of the distribution of money, power, and resources at the global, national, and local level, which in turn depends on the policies adopted in each context (Carmona and Parra 2015). In simple terms, this criterion seeks to understand "the causes of the causes," since these factors are often the fundamental sources of problems or differences in health. Likewise, the analysis of the influence of health promotion accompanied by behavioral changes that can modify the impact of environmental, social, and economic factors is proposed (Acero et al. 2013). As can be seen, the transformation of the concept of health permeated the different areas of knowledge that, in the case of the phenomenon of addictions, enriched the explanation of variations in substance consumption, by facilitating the inclusion of individual and behavioral factors, context in which people operate, from the closest to the most distal (Tse et al. 2016).

Therefore, the so-called ecological-integrative model for addiction care corresponds to a holistic approach that recognizes the complexity of the factors that contribute to drug consumption, based on the interrelationships and interdependencies of the sociocultural, biological and behavioral system that they converge in a complementary perspective of variables that can increase or decrease the risk of using psychoactive substances (Fernández et al. 2022). From the perspective of prevention, this allows us to design strategies that address not only individual needs, but are based on the conditions, needs, interests, social and environmental resources that can promote healthy lifestyles free of addictions. At the same time, with the recognition that prevention is part of a social and educational process, strategies are developed by context, which is defined as the set of circumstances that surround or condition an event in a defined scenario, where the meaning of behaviors, such as drug use, acquires specific connotations. The above gives rise to differentiated preventive actions, aimed at family, school, work, recreational, and community matters.

It can be seen then that this approach highlights the importance of a comprehensive and collaborative approach, recognizing the importance of treating the phenomenon with the participation of multiple sectors of society. It seeks to prevent the initial use of psychoactive drugs, as well as promote mental health, coping skills, and foster healthy interpersonal relationships, including friendships, family, and relationships. By merging these aspects, the ecological model offers a more complete vision, accepting that there is no single solution and that a multi-pronged approach is essential for its successful prevention and long-term treatment.

From Theoretical Models to Evidence-Based Prevention Programs

With the knowledge obtained from the maturation of the aforementioned explanatory models, it has been possible to understand increasingly better the biological, psychological, and sociocultural characteristics that modulate the initiation and maintenance of substance consumption of one person with respect to another. The above has helped to identify critical points in the addiction cycle, to develop strategies that address specific risk factors and define consistent methods to influence contexts, circumstances, and behaviors that favor protective factors. Thus, as part of the process to effectively address this public health issue, the transition must be made from theory to the design of drug use prevention programs.

A preventive program is the organized, coherent, and integrated set of actions that are based on a conceptual framework of reference, with the purpose of avoiding the appearance or incidence of the problem to which it is directed, in a specific population, for which it has a proven method and tools that allow the model to operate in large-scale scenarios (Fernández et al. 2022; Castro et al. 2015). In this sense and under a logic that takes into account quality standards, theoretical principles, and methodological guidelines that guarantee rigor and best practices agreed upon among leading organizations in the prevention of the use of psychoactive drugs, for preventive programs to be effective they must contemplate the next (European Monitoring Center for Drugs and Drug Addiction 2011; Cooperation Program between Latin America and the European Union on Drug Policies 2014; United Nations Office on Drugs and Crime 2018):

- Promote protective factors and reduce risk factors or their influence.
- Consider substances, both legal and illegal, and all forms of consumption.
- Contain skill strategies to address the offering of substances, reinforce personal commitment against their use, and increase social competence.
- Include interactive methods, such as opinion forums and not just teaching techniques.
- Have components that include parents or guardians, to reinforce the learning of girls, boys, adolescents, and young people, regarding the reality of drug consumption and its harmful effects, in order to generate family debate and reflection of the position that they adopt regarding substance use.
- Operate long term, from the first years of development and school cycles, with repeated interventions to reinforce the original preventive goals.
- Include media campaigns and policy changes, such as new rules and laws that restrict access to alcohol, tobacco, or other drugs, and which are more effective when accompanied by interventions in the family and at school.
- Strengthen norms against consumption in all prevention areas, including the family, school, and community.
- Adapt to each specific community to address the specific nature of the psychoactive substance abuse problem therein.

- The higher the risk in the target population, the more intensive preventive efforts should be and the earlier they should be initiated.
- Be specific to the age of the participants, appropriate to their period of development, and sensitive to cultural diversity.
- Be cost-effective.

In addition to the above, it must be taken into account that, according to the number and type of variables, as well as the relationship between them, theories have emerged that support preventive programs and offer different perspectives to address this public health challenge including (Fernández et al. 2022):

(a) Partial theories or theories based on few components. They focus on specific aspects of addiction, such as the influence of the environment and behavioral models on the acquisition of drug consumption habits. Some examples are biological, health belief, social learning, psychological, intrapersonal, family-based, and stress coping theories.
(b) Stage and evolutionary theories. They recognize that the addiction process varies over time and preventive programs must be adapted to its different stages. In this case, the model of stages of change is included, of the process of reaffirmation of young people, of maturity regarding drug consumption, of illness of psychosocial development of dependence on psychoactive substances, and of primary socialization.
(c) Integrative theories. It encompasses a broader range of factors, from individual to social and environmental. Among others, the theory of social learning, self-sufficiency, social development, risk or problem behaviors, lifestyles and risk factors, self-control and triadic influence are considered. Additionally, there are integrative theories for specific substances, such as self-determination, in the context of drug abuse prevention.
(d) Comprehensive and sequential theories of the phases of psychoactive consumption. They focus on a deep understanding of the motivations behind drug use and identify the stages of initiation and progression of consumption: phase of predisposition, knowledge, experimentation and initiation of consumption, consolidation of use to abuse and dependence, of abandonment or maintenance, of relapses.

In the case of Mexico, the previously mentioned background, enriched with the analysis of information on epidemiological trends in substance use in the national territory; the accumulated learning, both from successful experiences and lessons learned from the challenges faced in our context; and the exchange of knowledge and good practices through international studies have allowed the development of preventive interventions based on the particular characteristics and needs of the Mexican population (Castro et al. 2015). In turn, the Mexican State recognizes that the prevention of addictions requires the combined efforts of the public and private sectors, and coordinated actions to optimize resources and obtain better results. That is why, in the first decade of the twenty-first century, the Ministry of Health, through the National Commission against Addictions (CONADIC), published a document that integrates information on preventive models in matters of addiction, which summarizes the inter-institutional efforts carried out in the country. The above, under the premise that the prevention of addictions concerns everyone and that, to make it increasingly better, it is necessary to support it with strategies whose methods, procedures, and techniques allow us to overcome initiatives based solely on ideologies and convictions, to give rise to the application of models susceptible to evaluation that promote improvement with objective elements and replicable evidence (CONADIC 2002). This compilation reported the proposals that were being applied in school, family, and community contexts, including: (1) model build your life without addictions; (2) preventive model of Youth Integration Centers (CIJ); (3) model for preventing the use of alcohol, tobacco, and other drugs in the workplace; (4) preventive model of psychosocial risks for minors, adolescents, and their families Chimalli-DIF; (5) addiction prevention education program; (6) substance abuse prevention program for fourth, fifth, and sixth grade primary school students, I want I can; (7) community model of psychosocial integration; (8) education model for life and work: waters with addictions; (9) Chimalli preventive model of psychosocial risks; (10) professionalized social intervention model; and (11) ECO2 preventive model. Subsequently, in a new effort to put the progress of prevention in the country into perspective, the intention of a group of researchers arose to analyze the information on the programs in force at that time (Castro et al. 2015). In this case, 14 programs were reported: (1) CIJ model and preventive program "To live without addictions"; (2) Chimalli preventive model of psychosocial risks; (3) ECO2 metamodel; (4) program I want, I can; (5) community intervention program to discourage social risks associated with drug use; (6) model program for the prevention of alcohol, tobacco, and drug use in workers and their families; (7) interactive workshops for health promotion; (8) community intervention program for sex workers, with a harm reduction approach (9); prevention of addictive behaviors through positive parenting to reduce antisocial behavior; (10) construct T; (11) leaving little traces in your life; (12) positive parenting model; (13) Alas community selective prevention system; and (14) Ámbar Interactive Center.

In general terms, most programs are based on reducing risk factors and strengthening protective factors, with a tendency towards universal prevention interventions, but incorporating selective actions for communities with higher risk, as scientific evidence has suggested.

In relation to the context, it is in the school environment where the greatest proportion of the efforts made are directed, mainly to girls, boys, adolescents, and teachers, based on the fact that educational environments represent the ideal setting to influence beliefs and behaviors about substances. However, strategies that combine actions in different contexts are also common, which is based on evidence that points to multi-component interventions to obtain better results, rather than isolated ones. Likewise, the contributions of the evolution of evidence in prevention science are notable, with the incorporation of models that consider actions for the development of parental skills. As can be seen, even with the differences in the programs, they all agree on the recommendation of using interventions supported by the best scientific evidence available.

Evaluation of Preventive Programs

Although currently there is no place for preventive and treatment strategies for drug use to be developed based on intuition or mere will, this is a result of the evolution of the approaches through which the phenomenon has been addressed of addictions and the paradigm shift, which promotes adopting explanatory models based on science and empirically contrasted research. In this sense, the evaluation of psychoactive consumption prevention programs acquires exceptional importance in the context of evidence-based practice. As already mentioned, this methodology is based on solid scientific data and seeks to ensure that the interventions and strategies implemented are effective. Thus, evaluation in the field of drug use prevention provides the necessary elements to determine if a program meets its objectives, if it is generating a positive impact, and if it is the best way to use available resources. By collecting and analyzing data on program performance and outcomes, informed decisions can be made regarding continuation, expansion, or adjustment. This ensures the meticulous allocation of resources and promotes continuous improvement in the quality of interventions, contributing to the knowledge of best practices in prevention and allowing programs to adapt and transform to be more effective over time. Program evaluation is essential to protect the health and well-being of communities, especially the most vulnerable groups, by providing a basis to address this challenge actively and supported by evidence.

Preventive programs must necessarily be developed with designs that include measurement and monitoring tools for evaluation in terms of diagnosis, processes, results, and impact. Nowadays, most models focus on evaluating attitudinal changes, increased skills of attendees, changes in risk perception, willingness to change in the community, and increase in protective factors. There are also examples where results and impact measurements have been carried out in reducing substance consumption and associated problems. As a result of these, some preventive content has been institutionalized within the school curriculum, with which assertive behaviors and social skills have been increased to efficiently and healthily face the challenges presented to students. Likewise, school programs have favored the strengthening of the relationship between teachers and students, as well as the increase in youth participation.

Numerous international organizations have repeatedly called for rigorous evaluation of substance use prevention programs, as an essential measure to address this global phenomenon. Instances such as the United Nations Office on Drugs and Crime (UNODC), and the World Health Organization (WHO), have spoken out on the importance of collecting data, carrying out research, and regularly evaluating the strategies implemented worldwide. These calls are based on the urgency of ensuring that resources are used more effectively and on the identification of best practices that, in turn, contribute to the formulation of stronger policies and the development of programs sensitive to the needs of the population. This is how evaluation becomes crucial, by allowing the measurement of the success and effectiveness of prevention initiatives, while at the same time making it easier to detect areas of opportunity and make adjustments to ensure their usefulness in reducing drug demand.

Preventive Program "To live without addictions"

Being an example of resilience and long-term sustainability, the preventive program To Live Without Addictions has endured over time and illustrates the integration of the information discussed above (CIJ 2022). The Program was developed by Youth Integration Centers, a civil association assimilated to the Mexican health sector that, with more than 50 years of experience in mental health and addiction care, has been adapting its proposal in parallel to the evolution of the theoretical perspectives to explain the use of psychoactive substances, while it has been enriched with the contributions of science, until integrating the version currently in operation. It should be noted that the strategy is good enough to allow improvements based on the evidence that emerges from the research. To live without addictions is aimed at strengthening protective factors and reducing the incidence of those associated with drug use in individuals, families, and communities, considering social interaction in multiple contexts. The interventions and activities are designed according to the characteristics, resources, and needs of the population, and incorporate a community approach whose purpose is coordination with individual and social actors in the health, educational, social, and labor sectors, to strengthen participation citizenship and community involvement in mental health issues.

The intervention model considers five contexts of care: school, work, health, community, and virtual, without leaving aside the family environment, since it is constituted as a transversal axis incorporated from any of the others, that is, interaction is always contemplated of people with their environment, particularly with the family. In addition to the context, the stage of development is taken as a reference, based on the age group, to mitigate the specific risk factors they face throughout the life cycle, as well as the conditions of vulnerability and epidemiological emergency that affect the development and use of psychoactive substances. The above delimits the level of strategies (universal, selective, or indicated) which, in turn, can be operated under face-to-face, distance, or mixed modalities. Regarding this matter in particular, it is worth mentioning that preventive interventions have reached a greater number of spaces and populations thanks to new technologies, virtual connection, and its potential to generate communication between different groups, at different times and in different areas. In this regard, research indicates that addiction prevention can be achieved through virtual education, through distance strategies, to promote the teaching-learning process of resources and protection skills (Córdoba-Quintero and Restrepo-Escobar 2018). That is why the Program has incorporated multiple technological resources to deliver virtual materials and interventions to different populations, with the aim of promoting discussion and reflection on the effects of drugs, the development of psychosocial skills and competencies to address risk factors associated with the consumption of psychoactive substances. That said, it should be noted that the transversal axes applicable to this preventive intervention are respect for human rights, the gender perspective and community participation, especially youth. Figure 1 presents the integration of these components schematically.

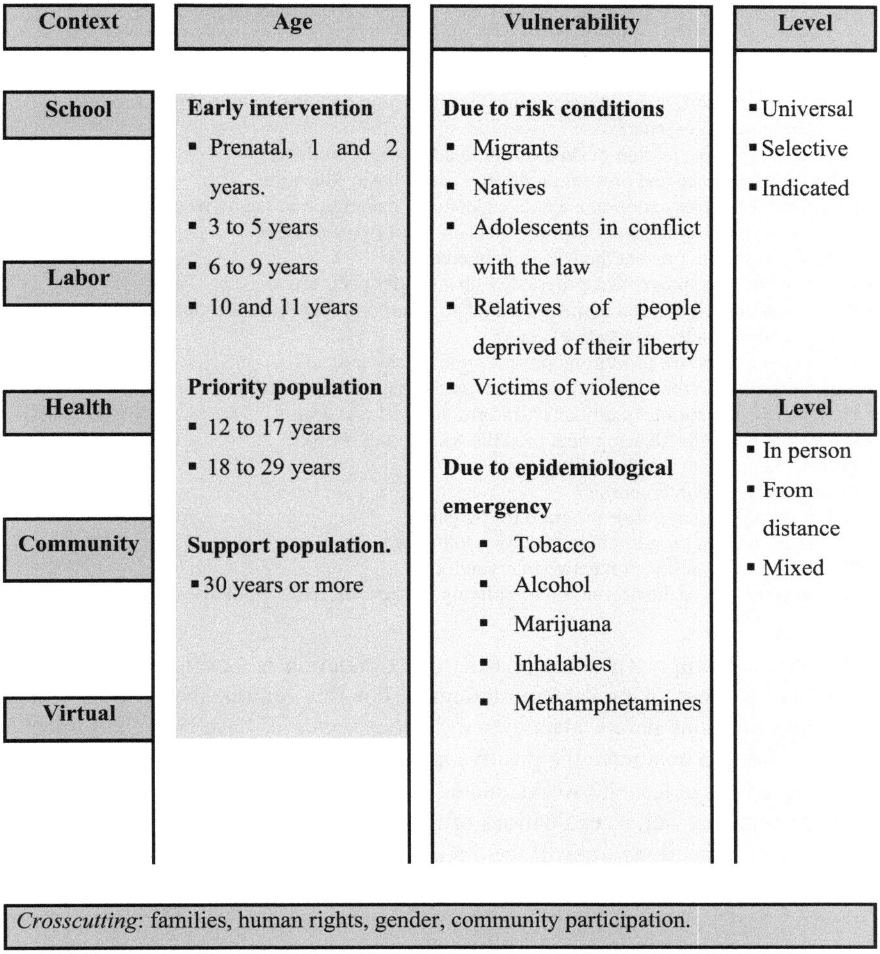

Fig. 1 Intervention model of the Preventive Program "To live without addictions"

As mentioned, addiction prevention programs must have a framework that allows understanding and explaining drug consumption and the dimensions, variables, and relationships to be considered; as well as define the strategies and mechanisms to achieve the desired changes, based on scientific evidence. Regarding the To Live Without Addictions program in particular, it is based on the following theoretical-methodological references: (a) public health approach; (b) model of risk and protective factors; (c) evolutionary perspective of human development; (d) social influence approach; (e) cognitive behavioral approach; (f) positive youth development model; (g) life skills; (h) social and emotional learning; (i) ecological/integrative model; (j) systemic approach and family-based theories; and (k) constructivist theories of learning.

Table 2 Evaluation studies of the Preventive Program of Youth Integration Centers

• Preventive program "To live without addictions."
• Prevention of drug use in the construction industry
• Promotion of assertive communication styles in coping with the supply of psychoactive substances in adolescents
• Intervention for prevention of drug use in middle school students
• School performance and prevention of drug use in basic education
• Program for the prevention of excessive alcohol consumption in young women
• Preventive family counseling: Comparative study of two strategies
• School program to prevent the use of amphetamines
• Violence and drug prevention program, with a gender perspective
• Prevention of violence and harmful alcohol consumption (psycho-educational orientation groups with a gender perspective)
• Efficacy of a selective prevention project aimed at adolescents
• Early intervention for Mexican preschool-aged girls and boys
• Preventive intervention "marijuana?: Inform yourself and decide."
• Preventive program "development of skills with young people."
• Preventive program with parents
• Online preventive interventions
• Universal prevention online program for parents
• Online prevention program indicated for adolescents
• "Socio-exciting" online preventive intervention
• Hybrid program for the prevention of bullying, addictions, and school disengagement

Finally, it is important to emphasize that evaluation is a critical component to ensure the success of preventive strategies. For this reason, the *To live without addictions* program and its adaptation to various scenarios have been the subject of study, in order to guarantee the positive impact of its implementation. This evaluative research has at least 80 works, including analysis of the reliability and validity of instruments, as well as evaluations of needs, processes, results, and impact (CIJ 2017). Table 2 mentions some of these studies.

Intersection Between Prevention Science and Public Policies

The formulation of public policies represents a fundamental pillar in the fight against addictions. To this end, prevention science, through research in psychology, sociology, neuroscience, and other disciplines, provides a deep understanding of the underlying factors that drive drug use; from individual aspects such as genetics and mental health, to social, economic, and cultural influences. This knowledge base becomes an invaluable resource for those responsible for formulating government guidelines.

Public policy has the power to translate scientific evidence into concrete actions. This involves the implementation of preventive strategies based on real data, such as educational programs, awareness campaigns, regulation of substance availability, and access to treatment and rehabilitation services.

By building a stable bridge from prevention science to public policy, information is translated into evidence-based state measures that can guide the allocation of resources, creation of laws, and implementation of preventive programs with a greater level of dissemination in a territory. Thus, collaboration between scientists, academics, and policymakers guarantees that the strategies adopted are relevant, effective, and adapted to the changing needs of society, thus contributing to the protection of public health, the reduction of drug consumption, and the mitigation of human suffering associated with the phenomenon of addictions. However, it is also important to highlight that the relationship between scientists and decision makers can be complex and is often influenced by political, economic, and cultural factors. Therefore, maintaining a constant and transparent dialogue between the research community, those responsible for public policies and society in general is essential to effectively address the consumption of psychoactive drugs and guarantee that strategies are effective and oriented toward well-being of everyone. Ultimately, this collaboration can make a difference in building healthier and more resilient societies.

In the Mexican context, a way to exemplify preventive efforts on a larger scale is the current National Addiction Prevention Strategy "Together for Peace" (ENPA 2019–2024), whose objective is to "impact the biopsychosocial determinants that prevent and reduce the use of psychoactive substances in boys, girls and youth for the construction of Peace, within the framework of human rights" (Secretary of Health 2022).

It is a collective commitment of the entire society, the three powers of the State, the three levels of government (federal, state, and municipal), the social and private sectors to change the traditional paradigm in terms of prevention of psychoactive substance consumption, towards a perspective that does not criminalize users, that treats people affected by addictions as a population worthy of the rights of protection, support, inclusion, and connection, to join a healthy and productive life in every sense. Among the lines of the previous statements, the contributions of the evolution of preventive approaches and the adoption of a comprehensive perspective that are aligned with the conventions on rights at a global level can be seen. The above, along with the virtue of being a far-reaching territorial effort, must necessarily be supported by practices based on the best scientific evidence available. Thus, a solid bridge will have been built that leads from science to public policy and from there to the well-being of individuals and societies, where evaluation appears as a crucial element in all stages.

The Future of Preventive Strategies

Based on the trends currently observed in drug consumption prevention interventions, the future is seen as a promising and constantly evolving field. Taking into account the available evidence, preventive models will have to be integrated into a broader public health framework, addressing not only substance use disorders, but also social determinants, such as inequality, poverty, and lack of access to education and mental health services. On this last point, it should be noted that the resolution presented by Mexico, on mental health and psychosocial support, before the United Nations General Assembly (2023), could also mark a milestone in the care of addictions. The above derives from the fact that the call to adopt strategies for the prevention of depression and suicide, as well as the improvement of emotional well-being, recognizes the close relationship between addictions and mental health. So, the promotion of healthy lifestyles and the prevention of drug use become basic components for future programs that seek to treat mental health problems and prevent them from worsening. Additionally, the resolution highlights the need to strengthen care services at all levels, which could guarantee effective support for those suffering from psychoactive use disorders, integrating prevention and treatment into a cohesive approach to mental health care. Together, these measures will contribute to a healthier future, where addressing drug use is intrinsically linked to the well-being of the population.

On the other hand, as we move into the twenty-first century, science and technology play a central role in improving interventions. In the coming years, neuroscientific and psychological research will provide greater understanding of the underlying mechanisms of substance abuse, which will drive the development of more specific and effective prevention strategies. In addition, the integration of technologies such as mobile applications, online platforms, and telemedicine will allow broader access to prevention and treatment services. Artificial intelligence and data analysis will help identify drug consumption patterns and predict trends more quickly, favoring the personalization of interventions; adapting them to the individual needs of people at risk, but also to a more efficient response from public health authorities. In summary, the future of strategies to prevent drug consumption is emerging as a multidimensional approach, based on evidence and oriented toward promoting the well-being and comprehensive health of communities. Advances in scientific understanding, technological innovation, and global collaboration will be the cornerstones of a more effective and compassionate approach to addressing the ongoing challenge that this phenomenon represents in society.

Conclusion

Throughout this chapter, the advances in the prevention of drug use have been discussed, a field in constant transformation, given the dynamic nature of the phenomenon of addictions. The evolution of approaches has moved from theory to action, shaping preventive programs that, within the framework of evidence-based practice, can result in positive outcomes for individuals and communities. Therefore, it is recommended that the actors involved, including scientists, academics, service operators, and decision makers, adopt prevention science, with its methodology and rigor, to design, implement, evaluate, and improve strategies aimed at preventing consumption of psychoactive substances.

Preventing drug use is a complex challenge that requires the collaboration of professionals, policymakers, and communities. There is no single solution, but scientific evidence and lessons learned from successful practice can guide the way to more effective strategies. Prevention is a constant and collective effort that, when supported by evidence, offers the opportunity for a healthier future for everyone. Addictions are a persistent phenomenon and prevention is an essential pillar.

References

Acero, M., Caro, I., Henao, L., Ruiz, E., & Sánchez, V. (2013). Determinantes Sociales de la Salud: postura oficial y perspectivas críticas. *Revista Facultad Nacional de Salud Pública*, 31(Suppl.1), 103-110. http://www.scielo.org.co/scielo.php?script=sci_arttext&pid=S0120-386X2013000400012

American Psychiatric Association. (1994). *Diagnostic and Statistical Manual of Mental Disorders* (4th ed.). Washington, DC: Author.

Asamblea General de las Naciones Unidas. (2023). *Resolución 77/L.77: "Salud mental y apoyo psicosocial"* (A/77/L.77). Sistema de Archivo de Documentos de las Naciones Unidas.

Arellanez, J. L. (2016). Consumo de drogas y respuestas al estrés migratorio entre los migrantes mexicanos que se dirigen a Estados Unidos. *Frontera norte*, *28*(56), 113-133.

Arellanez, J.L., Díaz, D.B., Wagner, F., & Pérez, V. (2004). Factores psicosociales asociados con el abuso y la dependencia de drogas entre adolescentes: Análisis bivariados de un estudio de casos y controles. *Salud Mental,* 27(3):54-64.

Becoña, I. (2002). *Bases científicas de la prevención de las drogodependencias*. Ministerio del Interior, Delegación del Gobierno para el Plan Nacional sobre Drogas.

Becoña, E. (1999). *Bases teóricas que sustentan los programas de prevención de drogas*. Universidad de Santiago de Compostela; Ministerio del Interior, Delegación del Gobierno para el Plan Nacional sobre Drogas.

Carmona, Z., & Parra, D. (2015). Determinantes sociales de la salud: un análisis desde el contexto colombiano. *Revista Salud Uninorte*, 31(3), 608-620. https://doi.org/10.14482/sun.31.3.7685

Castro, M. E., Llanes, J., Amador, N.G., Villatoro, J. & Medina-Mora, M.E. (2015). Capítulo 7. México. La Prevención del Consumo de Drogas en México. En A. Pérez Gómez, J. Mejía Trujillo, & B. Becoña Iglesia (Eds.), *De la prevención y otras historias: historia y evolución de la prevención del consumo de alcohol y drogas en América Latina y en Europa*. (114—131). California-Edit.

Castro, M.E., & Llanes, J. (2001). Estudio nacional del consumo de drogas en la población usuaria de la Preparatoria Abierta. En M. E. Medina-Mora (Coord.). *Observatorio epidemiológico en drogas, El fenómeno de las adicciones en México* (pp. 33-42). Secretaría de Salud, Consejo Nacional contra las Adicciones.

Castro, M.E. (1990). Indicadores de riesgo para el consumo problemático de drogas en jóvenes estudiantes, aplicación en investigación y atención primaria dentro del plantel escolar. *Salud pública de México,* 32(5): 298-308.

Centros de Integración juvenil, A.C. (2023). *Reporte del Sistema de Información Epidemiológica del Consumo de Drogas. Consumo de drogas en solicitantes de tratamiento en Centros de Integración Juvenil. Consumidores de Drogas Ilícitas. Segundo semestre del 2022.* CIJ. http://www.cij.gob.mx/programas/Investigacion/Epidemiologica.asp

Centros de Integración Juvenil, A.C. (2022). Programa Preventivo "*Para vivir sin adicciones*".

Centros de Integración Juvenil, A.C. (2019). *Estudio Básico de Comunidad Objetivo 2018. Introducción General.* http://www.cij.gob.mx/ebco2018-2024/Introduccion.html

Centros de Integración Juvenil, A.C. (2017). *Investigación Evaluativa*. http://www.cij.gob.mx/programas/Investigacion/Evaluativa.asp

Centros de Integración Juvenil. (2015). *Prevención del consumo de drogas en CIJ*. México: Centros de Integración Juvenil.

Consejo Nacional Contra las Adicciones. (2002). *Modelos Preventivos*. Serie Planeación. CONADIC, SS. ISBN 970-721-136-9. http://www.uade.inpsiquiatria.edu.mx/pagina_contenidos/libros/modelos_preventivos.pdf

Córdoba-Quintero, L. F., & Restrepo-Escobar, S. M. (2018) E-salud: Prevención del consumo de sustancias psicoactivas mediante la educación virtual. *Revista Colombiana de Ciencias Sociales*, 9(2), 362-382. https://doi.org/10.21501/22161201.2516

Córdova, A., Rodríguez, S., & Díaz, D.B. (2010). Bienestar subjetivo y calidad de vida en jóvenes usuarios y no usuarios de drogas. *Revista Intercontinental de Psicología y Educación*, 12(2), 147-162.

Degenhardt, L., Charlson, F., Ferrari, A., Santomauro, D., Erskine, H., Mantilla-Herrara, A., & Vos, T., et al. (2018). The global burden of disease attributable to alcohol and drug use in 195 countries and territories, 1990–2016: A systematic analysis for the Global Burden of Disease Study 2016. *The Lancet Psychiatry*, *5*(12), 987-1012. https://doi.org/10.1016/S2215-0366(18)30337-7

De La Guardia Gutiérrez, M. A., & Ruvalcaba Ledezma, J. C. (2020). La salud y sus determinantes, promoción de la salud y educación sanitaria. *Journal of Negative and No Positive Results*, *5*(1), 81-90. https://doi.org/10.19230/jonnpr.3215

Díaz N., D.B., Arellanez, J.L., Pérez, V., & Wagner, F. (2009). Correlatos psicosociales de involucramiento en el uso de drogas entre jóvenes mexicanos. *Revista Médica del Instituto Mexicano del Seguro Social, 47* (Supl. 1), S13-S20.

Díaz Negrete, B., & García Aurrecoechea, R. (2008). Factores psicosociales de riesgo de consumo de drogas ilícitas en una muestra de estudiantes mexicanos de educación media. *Revista Panamericana de Salud Pública*, 24, 223-232.

Fernández, C., Carrillo, M., & León, B. (2022). Modelos de prevención de adicciones basados en evidencias científicas. *Adicciones El creciente desafío* (pp. 253-281) Cátedra de Investigación Dr. Jorge Larrea Espinosa en Educación en Adicciones.

García Aurrecoechea, V. R., Rodríguez Kuri, S. E., Córdova Alcaráz, A. J., & Fernández Cáceres, M. D. C. (2016). Diagnóstico macrosocial de riesgo del consumo de drogas en México. *Acta de investigación psicológica*, *6*(3), 2516-2526. https://doi.org/10.1016/j.aipprr.2016.11.005

Griffin, K. W., & Botvin, G. J. (2010). Evidence-based interventions for preventing substance use disorders in adolescents. *Child and Adolescent Psychiatric Clinics of North America*, *19*(3), 505-526. https://doi.org/10.1016/j.chc.2010.03.005

Guyatt G., Cairns J., Churchill D., et al. (1992). Evidence-based medicine: A new approach to teaching the practice of medicine. *JAMA*, 268(17), 2420–2425. https://doi.org/10.1001/jama.1992.03490170092032

Harrop, E., & Catalano, R. F. (2016). Evidence-based prevention for adolescent substance use. *Child and adolescent psychiatric clinics*, *25*(3), 387-410. https://doi.org/10.1016/j.chc.2016.03.001

Hoffmann, T., & Glasziou, P. (2016). Bringing shared decision making and evidence-based practice together. *Shared Decision Making in Health Care*. Oxford University Press. https://doi.org/10.1093/acprof:oso/9780198723448.003.0039

Hopenhayn, M (2002). Prevenir en drogas: enfoques integrales y contextos culturales para alimentar buenas practicas (Serie: Políticas Sociales). Comisión Económica para America Latina y el Caribe (CEPAL). https://repositorio.cepal.org/server/api/core/bitstreams/25de1a2c-f9f8-4faf-9a0b-6b143b06831c/content

Instituto Nacional de Psiquiatría Ramón de la Fuente Muñiz; Instituto Nacional de Salud Pública, Comisión Nacional contra las Adicciones & Secretaría de Salud. (2017a) *Encuesta Nacional de Consumo de Drogas, Alcohol y Tabaco 2016-2017: Reporte de Drogas*. Villatoro-Velázquez J.A., Reséndiz-Escobar, E., Mujica-Salazar, A., Bretón-Cirett, M., Cañas-Martínez, V., Soto-Hernández, I., Fregoso-Ito, D., Fleiz-Bautista, C., Medina-Mora ME., Gutiérrez-Reyes, J., Franco-Núñez, A., Romero-Martínez, M. & Mendoza-Alvarado, L. Ciudad de México, México: INPRFM.

Instituto Nacional de Psiquiatría Ramón de la Fuente Muñiz; Instituto Nacional de Salud Pública, Comisión Nacional contra las Adicciones & Secretaría de Salud. (2017b). *Encuesta Nacional de Consumo de Drogas, Alcohol y Tabaco 2016-2017: Reporte de Alcohol*. Villatoro-Velásquez J. A., Reséndiz Escobar, E., Mujica Salazar, A., Bretón-Cirett, M., Cañas-Martínez, V., Soto-Hernández, I., Fregoso-Ito, D., Fleiz-Bautista, C., Medina-Mora ME., Gutiérrez-Reyes, J., Franco-Núñez, A., Romero-Martínez, M. & Mendoza-Alvarado, L. Ciudad de México, México: INPRFM.

Instituto Nacional de Psiquiatría Ramón de la Fuente Muñiz; Instituto Nacional de Salud Pública, Comisión Nacional Contra las Adicciones & Secretaría de Salud. (2017). *Encuesta Nacional de Consumo de Drogas, Alcohol y Tabaco 2016-2017: Reporte de Tabaco*. Reynales-Shigematsu L. M, Zavala-Arciniega L., Paz-Ballesteros W. C., Gutiérrez-Torres D. S., García-Buendía J. C., Rodríguez-Andrade M. A., Gutiérrez-Reyes, J., Franco-Núñez, A., Romero-Martínez, M. & Mendoza-Alvarado, L. Ciudad de México, México: INPRFM.

Jenicek M., (1997). Epidemiology, evidenced-based medicine, and evidence-based public health. *Journal of epidemiology, 7*(4), 187–197. https://doi.org/10.2188/jea.7.187

Leaf, P. J. (1999). A system of care perspective on prevention. *Clinical Psychology Review, 19*(4), 403-413. https://doi.org/10.1016/S0272-7358(98)00086-5

Lhachimi, S., Bala, M., & Vanagas, G. (2016). Evidence-Based Public Health. *BioMed research international, 2016*, 5681409. https://doi.org/10.1155/2016/5681409

Lerner, R. (2005). *Promoting positive youth development: Theoretical and empirical bases*. Institute for Applied Research in Youth Development, Tufts University. https://lifehouseduluth.org/wp-content/uploads/2015/02/Positive-Youth-Development.pdf

Mangrulkar L., Whitman C. & Posner M. (2001). *Enfoque de Habilidades para la Vida para un desarrollo saludable de niños y adolescentes*. OPS. División de Promoción y Protección de la Salud. Programa de Salud Familiar y Población. Washington, D.C.: Fundación Kellogg.

Medina-Mora, M.E., Cravioto, P., Villatorio, J., Fleiz, C., Galván, F., & Tapia, R. (2003). Consumo de drogas entre adolescentes: Resultados de la Encuesta Nacional de Adicciones, 1998. *Salud Pública de México 45* (supl.1): S16-S25

Ministerio de Educación de la Nación. (2009). *Prevención del consumo problemático de drogas desde el lugar del adulto en la comunidad educativa*. http://www.bnm.me.gov.ar/giga1/documentos/EL001387.pdf

Moscoso, A.J., & Titto O.M. (2015). *Problemáticas de las drogas. Orientaciones Generales. Prevención del uso indebido de drogas*. https://www.unodc.org/documents/bolivia/Prev_Problematica_de_las_drogas.pdf

Nevárez Sida, A., Carreón Rodríguez, V. G., & Bergman, M. (2022). Socioeconomic factors associated with drug consumption in Mexico. *Journal of Addictive Diseases, 40*(1), 12-18. https://doi.org/10.1080/10550887.2021.1919486

Nawi, A. M., Ismail, R., Ibrahim, F., Hassan, M. R., Manaf, M. R. A., Amit, N., & Shafurdin, N. S. (2021). Risk and protective factors of drug abuse among adolescents: a systematic review. *BMC public health, 21*(1), 1-15. https://doi.org/10.1186/s12889-021-11906-2

Nazar, A., Tapia, R., Villa, A., León, G., Medina-Mora, M.E., & Salvatierra, B. (1994). Factores asociados al consumo de drogas en adolescentes de áreas urbanas de México. *Salud Pública de México* 36(6): 646-654.

Newcomb, M.D., & Locke, T. (2005). Health, Social, and Psychological Consequences of Drug Use and Abuse. *Epidemiology of Drug Abuse*. https://doi.org/10.1007/0-387-24416-6_4

Newhouse, R. P., & Spring, B. (2010). Interdisciplinary evidence-based practice: Moving from silos to synergy. *Nursing outlook, 58*(6), 309-317. https://doi.org/10.1016/j.outlook.2010.09.001

Observatorio Europeo de Drogas y Toxicomanías (2011). *European drug prevention quality standards. A manual for prevention professionals*. EMCDDA.

Pérez, V. & Díaz, D.B. (2011). *Relación entre la percepción de la violencia social y el uso de drogas en jóvenes estudiantes de educación media. Informe de Investigación 11-10*. Dirección de Investigación y Enseñanza. Subdirección de Investigación. Centros de Integración Juvenil.

Programa de Cooperación entre América Latina y la Unión Europea en Políticas sobre Drogas (2014). *Calidad y evidencia en reducción de la demanda de drogas. Marco de referencia para la acreditación de programas*. Madrid: Copolad, Entidad de Coordinación y Ejecución.

Robinson, S. M., & Adinoff, B. (2016). The classification of substance use disorders: Historical, contextual, and conceptual considerations. *Behavioral Sciences*, *6*(3), 18. https://doi.org/10.3390/bs6030018

Rodríguez-Kuri, S. E., García-Aurrecoechea, R., Benítez-Villa, J. L., & Fernández-Cáceres, C. (2019). Diagnosis of macrosocial risks of drug use in Mexican municipalities. *Salud mental*, *42*(1), 5-12. https://doi.org/10.17711/sm.0185-3325.2019.002.

Rodríguez, S., Díaz, D.B., Garcia, S., Guerrero, A., & Lucio, E. (2007) Capacidad predictiva de la Teoría de la Conducta Planificada en la intención y uso de drogas ilícitas entre estudiantes mexicanos. *Salud Mental* 30(1): 68-81.

Rodríguez, S., Arellanez, J.L., Díaz, D.B., & González, D. (1998). *Ajuste psicosocial y consumo de drogas*. Centros de Integración Juvenil, Informe de investigación 97-27. México.

Salinas, E., Cabrera, J. Domínguez, A., Zapata R., Díaz-Negrete, D.B., Quinanilla, et al. (1997). Riesgos macrosociales de farmacodependencia a nivel municipal y red estratégica de atención en México. Plan Rector Institucional 1998-2000. *Riesgos macrosociales de farmacodependencia a nivel municipal y red estratégica de atención en México. Plan Rector Institucional 1998-2000* (pp. 217-217).

Sánchez Hoil, A., Andueza Pech, M. G., Santana Carvajal, A. M., Hoil Santos, J. J., & CuFarfán López, J. (2017). Características sociodemográficas y perfil de consumo de tabaco y drogas en estudiantes de dos universidades de México. *Revista biomédica*, *28*(1), 11-27.

Sánchez, M. & Velasco C., (2017). El modelo de Leavell y Clark como marco descriptivo dentro de las investigaciones sobre el virus de la Hepatitis B en niños con infección por VIH/SIDA del grupo de investigación gastrohnup de la universidad del valle de Cali, Colombia. *Revista Gastrohnup* 15(3), S6-S9.

Secretaría de Salud (2022).Estrategia Nacional de Prevención de Adicciones. "Juntos por la Paz". 2018-2024.

Smith, R., & Rennie, D. (2014). Evidence-based medicine—an oral history. *Jama*, *311*(4), 365-367. https://doi.org/10.1001/jama.2013.286182

Substance Abuse and Mental Health Services Administration (SAMHSA). (2019). *Substance Misuse Prevention for Young Adults*. https://store.samhsa.gov/sites/default/files/d7/priv/pep19-pl-guide-1.pdf

Tavera, S. & Martínez, M., (s/f). *Prevención de las adicciones y promoción de conductas saludables para una nueva vida. Guía para el promotor de "Nueva Vida"*. Consejo Nacional Contra las Adicciones. http://docs.saludchiapas.gob.mx/transparencia/pot/f01/F01_461.pdf

Tse, S., Zhu, S., Yu, C. H., Wong, P., y Tsang, S. (2016). An ecological analysis of secondary school students' drug use in Hong Kong: A case-control study. *The International journal of social psychiatry*, 62(1), 31–40. https://doi.org/10.1177/0020764015589132

Uhl, G. R., Koob, G. F., & Cable, J. (2019). The neurobiology of addiction. *Annals of the New York Academy of Sciences*, *1451*(1), 5-28. https://doi.org/10.1111/nyas.13989

United Nations Office on Drugs and Crime [UNODC]. (2023). *World Drug Report*. https://www.unodc.org/unodc/en/data-and-analysis/world-drug-report-2023.html

United Nations Office on Drugs and Crime [UNODC]. (2018). *International Standards on Drug Use Prevention*. https://www.unodc.org/documents/prevention/UNODC-WHO_2018_prevention_standards_E.pdf

Villatoro, J., Hernández. I., Hernández, H., Fleiz, C., Blanco, J., & Medina-Mora, M.E. *Encuestas de consumo de drogas en estudiantes III*, 1991-2003. Secretaría de Educación Pública, Instituto Nacional de Psiquiatría, disco compacto, México, 2004.

José Luis Benítez Villa is Master's and PhD in Health Sciences specialized in epidemiology, from the National Autonomous University of Mexico (UNAM). Head of the International Relations Department in Centros de Integración Juvenil (CIJ). Member of the CONAHCyT's National System of Researchers (SNII). National Chapter's Advisory Committee Member and leader trainer of the International Society of Substance Use Professionals (ISSUP).

Carmen Fernández-Cáceres Bachelor's degree in Psychology from Universidad Anáhuac, Master's in Family Therapy from the Latin American Institute of Family Studies (ILEF), and Doctorate in Psychoanalysis and Family and Couples Therapy. Member of the Editorial Board of the Journal of Substance Use and the Executive Editor of the International Journal of Addiction Research. She is currently the General Director of Centros de Integración Juvenil (CIJ), the General Coordinator of the "Dr. Jesús Kumate Rodríguez" Chair in Addictions, and the Academic Coordinator of the Master's in Addiction Management program, both at Universidad Anáhuac.

Substance Abuse and Addiction in Türkiye: Prevention, Policies, and Future Recommendations

Murat Yıldırım, Fatma Celik Tanrıverdi, and Muhammed Berat Geçit

Country Context

Situated at the crossroads of Europe and Asia, Türkiye acts as a bridge between Eastern and Western cultures, showcasing a diverse blend of traditions. With a population exceeding 86.1 million as of March 13, 2024, Türkiye stands as one of the most populous countries in its region. Its landscape ranges from bustling cities to tranquil coastlines and impressive mountains. Türkiye embraces and values religious and cultural diversity, with Islam as the predominant faith. Its strategic position between Europe and Asia makes it a key player in the globe. From ancient ruins to bustling markets, Türkiye offers a rich tapestry of experiences for visitors, blending modernity with heritage in a captivating fusion of sights and sounds.

M. Yıldırım (✉)
Department of Psychology, Faculty of Science and Letters, Agri Ibrahim Cecen University, Ağrı, Türkiye
e-mail: muratyildirim@agri.edu.tr

F. C. Tanrıverdi
Department of Psychology, Faculty of Science and Letters, Duzce University, Düzce, Türkiye
e-mail: fatmacelik@duzce.edu.tr

M. B. Geçit
Department of Philosophy and Religious Sciences, Ataturk University, Erzurum, Türkiye
Turkish Green Crescent Foundation, Ağrı, Türkiye

A. Pérez-Gómez, J. Mejía-Trujillo (eds.), *Drug Abuse Prevention*, Advances in Mental Health and Addiction, https://doi.org/10.1007/978-3-031-99621-4_6

Introduction

Türkiye's climate and soil conditions are well-suited for the cultivation of addictive plants such as hemp and poppy. These crops have been cultivated in our country for many years, and the specific cultivation areas for hemp have been defined with Law No. 2313. Presently, the Ministry of Agriculture and Forestry oversees and permits hemp cultivation (Taşlıgil & Şahin, 2018).

Throughout its historical development, Türkiye has been involved in the production and export of drugs. Particularly, after the First World War, there was a notable increase in this activity (Köknel, 1976). Sadly, substance abuse remains a pressing issue in Türkiye. While the number of deaths related to substance abuse has decreased compared to previous years, there is still a significant interest in these substances. In 2022, among the deaths attributed to substance abuse, 140 were linked to methamphetamine, 67 to heroin, and 46 to ecstasy. Notably, in 2020 and 2019, the majority of substance-related deaths were associated with methamphetamine (Türkiye Uyuşturu Raporu, 2023, p.94). The rising use of methamphetamine underscores the need for increased social awareness and a concerted effort by institutions to curb the demand for this substance. This section will delve into the historical developments and changes related to drugs in Türkiye since the time of the Ottoman Empire.

Policies and Strategies for the Prevention of Addiction in Türkiye

Following the transition to the Presidential Administration System in Türkiye in 2018, a series of institutional regulations were implemented. These changes involved revisions to the legislation related to addiction. Importantly, Presidential Decree No. 2019/2 played an important role in reconstituting the High Council for Combating Addiction (BMYK). This council welcomed the participation of key ministers, including those from the Ministries of Justice, Family, Labour and Social Services, Environment and Urbanisation, Youth and Sports, Treasury and Finance, Interior, National Education, Health, Agriculture and Forestry, Trade, Transport and Infrastructure, and the Deputy Chairman of the Presidential Health and Food Policies Board. The primary focus of this restructured council, in close collaboration with relevant ministries, has been on addressing substance addictions and abuse, including drugs, alcohol, and tobacco, as well as behavioural addictions such as gambling and technology addiction (Türkiye Drug Report, 2023).

Under the directive of the High Council, and with the Ministry of Health, provincial coordination boards have been established across all 81 provinces of Türkiye, operating under the chairmanship of the respective governor. These boards are responsible for reporting on addiction-related activities, conducting assessments, and delivering results every 6 months to the UNHCR, which subsequently compiles and publishes an annual report for public scrutiny. Additionally, these boards stand ready to provide support to public institutions in their activities to combat addiction. Furthermore, it is important to note that Circular No. 2017/23 has been rescinded (Türkiye Drug Report, 2023).

Legal Regulations Concerning Addictive Substances in Türkiye

Historically, the legal framework of Türkiye in addressing addictive substances has undergone a series of significant developments. In 1906, the country took its initial step in controlling the impact of cocaine by instituting a ban on its importation. Subsequently, more comprehensive legislation was introduced in 1917, representing an important step in regulating the use of addictive substances beyond the domain of healthcare. Importantly, this legislative milestone incorporated punitive measures aimed at curbing illicit drug-related activities (Tekin, 2005).

Within the Turkish Penal Code, Articles 403—408 are specifically dedicated to the field of "drug offences". These provisions articulate stringent penalties, encompassing imprisonment and financial fines, targeting individuals engaged in a spectrum of drug-related activities, all in the absence of the requisite licenses. Activities falling under scrutiny include the transportation, possession, processing of raw materials, manufacturing, sale, purchase, and facilitation of the trade or acquisition of drugs (Legislation, n.d.).

Law No. 1369 on narcotic drugs, initially enacted in 1928, and subsequently augmented by a decree dated 15.02.1931, focuses on the conditions surrounding the possession, processing, and trade of narcotic substances. It sanctioned the sale of drugs in pharmacies for medicinal purposes, subject to authorization from the Ministry of Health and Social Welfare. However, it restricted the use of substances containing more than 20% cocaine and over 10% morphine exclusively to pharmacists holding the approval of the relevant Ministry. Furthermore, the law stipulated that pharmacies exceeding the designated limits of narcotic substances would face the revocation of their license for importing such substances from abroad (Law No Official Gazette. 1369, 1928). Furthermore, the law on narcotic drugs, under Article 3, takes an unequivocal stance against the cultivation of cannabis for the production of marijuana, the preparation of substances for consumption, and their import, export, and sale. It also encompassed provisions from the previously mentioned Law No. 1369 (Law No Official Gazette. 1369, 1928).

Additionally, the law empowers customs officers to confiscate narcotic substances illicitly entering the country without the appropriate authorization. These seized substances are subsequently entrusted to the custody of the public prosecution office. Over time, amendments have been introduced to various articles. Importantly, a 2003 revision to Article 21 specified that some of the confiscated substances would be utilized in training dogs for drug detection purposes.

Furthermore, Article 23 witnessed modifications, such as the May 23, 1990 amendment under Article 3652/1, which mandated that the cultivation of hemp must be conducted under the supervision of the Ministry of Agriculture, Forestry, and Rural Affairs. Growing cannabis without permission from the Ministry is strictly prohibited, and those caught cultivating hemp or marijuana plants face penalties (Law No. 3652, 2020). Under this law, police officers are granted the authority to close down establishments involved in the possession, production, sale, or distribution of narcotic drugs, under orders from their superiors. Moreover, the police have the power to arrest individuals engaged in narcotic substance activities (Law No. 3652, 2020).

Initiatives for Combating Addiction in Türkiye

a. *High Council for Combating Addiction*

On December 9, 2017, the High Council for Combating Addiction was established through Prime Ministry Circular No. 2017/23, with the Deputy Prime Minister as its chairperson, and the participation of 11 ministers. The primary aim of the High Council for Combating Addiction (BMYK) is to mitigate exposure society to all forms of addictive substances and behaviours. It also strives to foster a society composed of individuals who are mentally, physically, and socially healthy. Subsequently, on February 14, 2019, Presidential Circular No. 2019/2 led to the reconstitution of the UNHCR, with the Vice President at the helm, and the involvement of 11 ministers and the Vice President of the Presidential Health and Food Policies Board (BMYK, 2023).

b. *Türkiye Addiction Fighting Training Program*

The Türkiye Addiction Fighting Training Program (TBM), which was developed by the Green Crescent, encompasses modules emphasizing preventive measures for healthy living to combat various forms of addiction. TBM represents a primary intervention program designed to educate children, young people, and society at large on the principles of healthy living. Since 2014, TBM has reached an approximate audience of 10 million students and 3 million adults annually, thanks to the efforts of 812 trainers (counsellors) and 33,389 facilitators, working in collaboration with the Ministry of National Education, public institutions, and the private sector (TBM, 2023). This program caters to various groups, including students from kindergarten to high school, parents, adults, and practitioners. Each group is provided with online and in-person access to addiction-related materials, comprising 18 modules. These modules include books, audiobooks, presentations, audio presentations, posters, 30-minute interactive videos, measurement tools, and brochures (Yoldaş & Demircioğlu, 2020, p. 76). To ensure efficacy, TBM conducts measurement and evaluation assessments for all modules. Consequently, the content of the program is systematically re-evaluated and updated. As of 2022, TBM stands as one of the most comprehensive addiction prevention programs in Türkiye, dedicated to raising awareness among individuals regarding the perils of addiction (TBM, 2023).

c. *Narkotim*

The primary aims of Narkotim, which was established by the General Directorate of Security (EGD) in 2014, is to thwart street-level drug offences within society in Türkiye. Under the auspices of the EGM Department of Combating Narcotic Crimes, Narkotim's professionalization efforts have extended across all provinces of Türkiye, enhancing the fight against drug demand. Since 2014, Narkotim has persistently engaged in operational activities targeting drug supply within venues like parks, school environments, and other locations conducive to drug trafficking (NARKOTIM, 2023).

d. *School Addiction Intervention Program*

School Addiction Intervention Program (OBM) has been implemented by 465 Guidance and Psychological Counselling Teachers (PCT) in schools across all 81 provinces of Türkiye since 2019, The OBM aims to deliver preventive interventions against tobacco, alcohol, addictive substance use, and technological addiction—experiences commonly faced by students. Developed in collaboration with the Ministry of National Education and the Green Crescent, OBM equips PCTs with the professional skills necessary to communicate effectively with students and acquire competencies in addiction intervention, including guiding at-risk students. OBM's cooperative efforts with PCTs involve identifying students vulnerable to addiction, evaluating their situations, conducting essential interventions, and closely monitoring progress through follow-up interviews. These interventions encompass informing students about the addiction process, conducting motivational interviews, strengthening family communication, and providing psychosocial support. OBM focuses on students in the experimentation or initial usage phase of drugs, aiming to prevent addiction within the school environment while preserving students' right to education (OBM, 2023).

e. *Green Crescent Life Skills Training Program*

Commencing in the 2021–2022 academic year, the Green Crescent Life Skills Education Programme (YYBE) was introduced in secondary schools across all provinces of Türkiye. Approximately 5000 students have been reached by 151 guidance counsellors implementing the program. The primary target audience comprises 7th-grade students, with additional support provided when these students transition to the 8th grade. YYBE seeks to educate students with a wide array of skills, including stress management, prevention of negative emotions, effective communication, critical thinking, decision-making, regulation of peer relationships, refusal skills against addiction, and protection against risky situations. The research highlights the efficacy of the program, emphasizing its emphasis on life skills, its substantial influence on enhancing students' substance use rejection skills, and its capacity to boost self-efficacy in resisting substance addiction. YYBE represents a school-based, protective, and empowering educational program that instils positive behavioural changes and habits in students, enabling them to safeguard themselves from adverse environments and situations that could lead to addiction (YYBE, 2023). In particular, YYBE was effective in enhancing life skills among students, by demonstrating higher life skills compared to those who did not undergo the program. The results indicated that the program successfully improved students' self-awareness, coping mechanisms for negative emotions, and critical thinking skills, while also enhancing their ability to refuse smoking (YYBE, 2023).

Rehabilitation Programs for Individuals Struggling with Addiction

a. *Alcohol and Substance Addicts Treatment Centre*

The first addiction treatment centre was founded in 1980 at Istanbul's Bakırköy Mental Health and Nervous Diseases Hospital. It was subsequently rebranded as the Alcohol and Drug Addicts Treatment Centre (AMATEM). Rehabilitation centres for addicts in Türkiye represent a crucial therapeutic milestone. AMATEM operates as an outpatient or inpatient facility, catering to individuals aged 18 and older with alcohol or substance use disorders. The centre was purposefully established to serve those struggling with alcohol and substance addiction, aiming to provide counselling, treatment, and rehabilitation services and prevent such addictions (AMATEM, 2023).

b. *Child and Adolescent Drug Addiction Treatment Centre*

In 1995, Bakırköy Prof. Dr Mazhar Osman Mental Health and Neurological Diseases Training and Research Hospital initiated a centre known as the Volatile Substances Research and Treatment Centre (UMATEM), with the backing of the Istanbul Governorship, aimed at separating the treatment processes for addicted adult and paediatric patients. Over time, this centre expanded its scope and was renamed the Child and Adolescent Substance Addiction Treatment Centre (ÇEMATEM), dedicated to individuals under the age of 18. The core objective of this treatment is not merely to help children overcome drug and alcohol addiction but also to prevent relapse and ensure their reintegration into society as healthy and productive individuals. To achieve this goal, the centre employs various treatment and therapy methods designed to strengthen both the family and the child, restore mental and physical well-being, and foster the development of a new lifestyle. Throughout the treatment and therapy process, a range of activities, including good morning meetings, group therapies, individual interviews and follow-up visits, Turkish and mathematics lessons, hobby sessions (such as crafts, art, and folklore), and age-appropriate sports activities, are provided to contribute to the healing process and facilitate rehabilitation. Additional measures, such as assignments within the service, reading sessions, and vocational training activities, are included to promote responsibility (Bakırköy, 2019 & Ögel, n.d.).

c. *Green Crescent Consultancy Centre*

In 2013, the Green Crescent broadened its services to include rehabilitation through a legal change. The Green Crescent Counselling Centre (YEDAM) was subsequently established in 2015. Initially, it functioned as a call centre, but since

2016, it has offered rehabilitation support to addicts and their families, providing free face-to-face counselling services as part of a pilot program in the Üsküdar district of Istanbul in Türkiye. Collaboration with various expert professionals, including psychologists, social workers, and public relations specialists, is a cornerstone of YEDAM's approach. Employees receive ongoing supervision support tailored to their respective areas of expertise. A total of 107 YEDAM centres operate in all 81 provinces of Türkiye and the Turkish Republic of Northern Cyprus (KKTC), offering services to individuals grappling with addiction and their families. These individuals can access free call centres and counselling services by dialling 115. In this context, counselling is extended to addicts, their families, and relatives to raise awareness about addiction and enhance their skills. Group counselling services are also available for adolescents, adults, and family members of addicted individuals. In cases where the addicted individual is unwilling to accept counselling, support is provided to those in the individual's immediate environment, with the ultimate aim of engaging the addicted individual in the treatment process and facilitating their healthy reintegration into society. In this regard, various activities are employed, including motivational interventions, professional development initiatives, support for reintegration into educational life, and skill development courses. To further support the YEDAM model, 24 working groups have been established, tasked with advancing the treatment of various addiction types, conducting scientific research, and fostering professional development among employees. Statistics from the Green Crescent Counselling Centre indicate that between 2016 and 2022, there were 28,764 initial applications, 548,859 calls to the counselling line, 113,855 interviews, 49,737 instances of social support services, and 450 social activities conducted (YEDAM, 2021).

d. *Rehabilitation Center for Dependent Patients*

The Tuzla Addicted Patients Rehabilitation Centre (BAHAR), situated within the Erenköy Mental and Neurological Diseases Training and Research Hospital in Istanbul, Türkiye, initiated its provision of rehabilitation services for addicts aged 18–25 on February 18, 2019. BAHAR represents Türkiye's first outpatient rehabilitation centre for adult addicted patients, featuring a personalized and structured module and a range of interdisciplinary services. To be eligible for admission to BAHAR centres, individuals must be voluntary, and substance-free, have completed their treatment, participated in basic psycho-educational addiction groups, and maintained their well-being for at least three weeks. These individuals undergo an assessment by the treatment team before being included in the program (BAHAR, 2023).

e. *Green Crescent Rehabilitation Centre*

In 2019, the Green Crescent Rehabilitation Centres introduced inpatient services, offered free of charge, with a strong commitment to safeguarding the confidentiality of addicted individuals. The Green Crescent Addiction Rehabilitation Centre (REHAB), accessible to individuals who have completed medical treatment and are drug-free, seeks to facilitate their reintegration into social life. A structured treatment program is implemented based on the type and severity of addiction and the socio-economic analysis of the individuals. Individuals can remain in the centre for a minimum of 3 months and a maximum of 1 months by the structured treatment program (REHAB, 2020).

Conclusion and Recommendations

Over time, Türkiye has engaged in a multifaceted effort to combat substance addiction, with various governmental and non-governmental organizations. This collaborative approach has led to effective addiction prevention strategies, including initiatives like YYBE implemented by Green Crescent. This approach includes various dimensions of the fight against addiction, thereby addressing the issue in a well-rounded manner. It appears that therapeutic rehabilitation centers for substance addicts may potentially demonstrate effectiveness. Furthermore, there is hope that intervention centres will improve, becoming as effective as rehabilitation centres, which could help reduce the number of addicts in the country.

When the efforts to combat drug abuse in Türkiye are reviewed, it is evident that there is a strong commitment from both the government and the state. They have established various institutions, regulations, laws, projects, and initiatives to effectively address this issue. The expectation is that as these institutions continue to expand, and as multidisciplinary teams within them grow, with more experts dedicated to their mission and improved professional development, these collective efforts will yield positive results in the ongoing fight against addiction.

The efforts of Türkiye to combat addiction have evolved into a multifaceted strategy. This strategy combines various approaches, including rehabilitation for addicts, preventive measures, and awareness campaigns to discourage addictive behaviours. To cope with this problem more effectively, future recommendations may include increased investment in research, improved coordination among government and non-governmental organizations, a stronger focus on education and community support, and enhanced mental health services. Early intervention strategies could further strengthen the nation's fight against addiction, leading to a healthier and more resilient society. Each of these recommendations is presented in detail below.

First, a critical aspect of tackling addiction is to gain a better understanding of its causes, patterns, and outcomes. Investing in research can help us comprehend evidence-based strategies and interventions related to substance abuse and addiction. More studies can shed light on the factors contributing to addiction and help identify high-risk populations. By dedicating resources to research, Türkiye can stay ahead of emerging challenges and refine its approach to addiction prevention and treatment.

Second, collaboration among various stakeholders is essential for a well-coordinated response to addiction. Government bodies, non-governmental organizations, healthcare providers, and community support groups must work together seamlessly. Establishing clear communication channels and sharing resources can improve efforts to combat addiction. This coordination ensures that support services are readily available and that no individual or community is left underserved.

Third, prevention is a key component of addiction control. Focusing on educational programs that raise awareness about the risks associated with substance abuse and addictive behaviours is crucial. Schools, community centres, and healthcare facilities can serve as platforms for disseminating information and providing support. Community-based initiatives, such as support groups and counselling services, play an essential role in helping individuals make informed choices and providing a safety net for those at risk.

Fourth, addiction often co-occurs with mental health issues. Enhancing mental health services not only helps in identifying and addressing underlying psychological factors contributing to addiction but also offers support for individuals in recovery. This includes access to counselling, therapy, and psychiatric care. By enhancing mental health services, Türkiye can effectively address the challenges of addiction and mental well-being.

Finally, identifying individuals at risk of addiction at an early stage is crucial. Implementing early intervention strategies can prevent the progression of addictive behaviours and improve recovery outcomes. Schools, healthcare providers, and community organizations should be equipped to recognize early signs of addiction and offer timely assistance. These approaches can assist people in getting support before their addiction becomes more severe.

In conclusion, by incorporating these recommendations into its addiction control efforts, Türkiye can work towards building a healthier and more resilient society. A better and well-coordinated approach that includes research, education, community support, mental health services, and early intervention strategies will contribute to more effective prevention and treatment of addiction and substance abuse.

References

Alcohol and Substance Addicts Treatment Centre [AMATEM]. (2023). AMATEM. October 09, 2023, from http://www.amatem.org/

Bakırköy (2019). ÇEMATEM. October 08, 2023, from https://bakirkoyruhsinireah.saglik.gov.tr/TR-346325/cematem.html#

Drug Report for 2023. (2023). Türkiye Uyuşturucu Raporu: Eğilimler ve Gelişmeler. September 05, 2023, from https://narkotik.pol.tr/kurumlar/narkotik.pol.tr/TUB%C4%B0M/Ulusal%20Yay%C4%B1nlar/2023_TURKIYE_UYUSTURUCU_RAPORU.pdf

Established by the General Directorate of Security [NARKOTIM]. (2023). Bağımlılıkla Mücadele Yüksek Kurulu. October 08, 2023, from https://bmyk.gov.tr/TR-73370/narkotim.html

Green Crescent Rehabilitation Centre [REHAB]. (2020). Yeşilay Rehabilitasyon Merkezleri (REHAB). October 01, 2023, from https://www.yesilay.org.tr/tr/yesilay-rehabilitasyon-merkezleri-rehab

Green Crescent Life Skills Training Program [YYBE]. (2023). Yeşilay Yaşam Becerileri Eğitim Programı (YYBE). October 08, 2023, from https://bmyk.gov.tr/TR-87192/yesilay-yasam-becerileri-egitim-programi-yybe.html

Green Crescent Consultancy Centre [YEDAM]. (2021). October 05, 2023, from https://www.yedam.org.tr/
High Council for Combating Addiction [BMYK]. (2023). September 16, 2023, from https://bmyk.gov.tr/
Köknel, Ö. (1976). İnsanlık Tarihi Boyunca Dünyada ve Türkiye'de Uyuşturucu Madde Sorunları, Gelişim Yayınları, İstanbul.
Law No Official Gazette. 1369 [1369 Sayılı Kanun Resmi Gazete]. (1928). Sempember 07, 2023, from https://www.resmigazete.gov.tr/arsiv/1074.pdf
Law No. 3652. (2020). September 10, 2023, https://www.mevzuat.gov.tr/mevzuat?MevzuatNo=2313&MevzuatTur=1&MevzuatTertip=3
Legislation. (n.d.). September 09, 2023, from https://www.mevzuat.gov.tr/mevzuatmetin/5.3.765.pdf
Ögel, K. (n.d.). "UMATEM'den ÇEMATEM'e: Bir İstanbul Öyküsü". October 08, 2023, from http://www.ogelk.net/makale/69-herkes-icin-not-defteri-umatem-den-cematem-e-bir-istanbul-oykusu-.html
Rehabilitation Center for Dependent Patients [BAHAR]. (2023). 08 October 2023, from https://bmyk.gov.tr/TR-69379/bagimli-hastalar-icin-rehabilitasyon-merkezi-bahar.html
School Addiction Intervention Program [OBM]. (2023). October 08, 2023, from https://bmyk.gov.tr/TR-69382/okulda-bagimliliga-mudahale-egitim-programi-obm.html
Taşlıgil, N., & Şahin, G. (2018). Tarihsel Süreçte Haşhaş (Papaver somniferum L.) ve Afyon.
Tekin, M. (2005). Cumhuriyet Döneminde Türkiye'de uyuşturucu madde kullanımı ile mücadele (1920-1940).
Türkiye Addiction Fighting Training Program [TBM]. (2023). October 08, 2023, from https://bmyk.gov.tr/TR-69381/turkiye-bagimlilikla-mucadele-egitim-programi-tbm.html
Yoldaş, C., & Demircioğlu, H. (2020). Madde kullanımı ve bağımlılığını önlemeye yönelik psikoeğitim programlarının incelenmesi. *Bağımlılık Dergisi*, *21*(1), 72-91.

Murat Yıldırım is currently working at the Department of Psychology at Agri Ibrahim Cecen University, Türkiye. His research mainly focuses on happiness, mental well-being, personality, emotions, and coping strategies.

Fatma Celik Tanriverdi is currently works at the Psychology Department, Duzce University. Fatma conducts research in the field of applied psychology, positive psychology, social psychology and psychoanalysis.

Muhammed Berat Geçit is currently working at Department of Philosophy and Religious Sciences, Ataturk University, Türkiye and areas of expertise are substance abuse, counseling, clinical psychology and psychology of religion.

United States National Substance Use Prevention: An Overview of Prior Campaigns and a View to the Future

William D. Crano, Eusebio M. Alvaro, and Jason T. Siegel

Country Context

The United States, located in North America, is a diverse and vibrant nation comprising 50 states, one federal district, and several territories. With a population of more than 330 million people, it is one of the most populous countries in the world. Its geography varies, ranging from the Rocky Mountains and deserts of the Southwest to the plains of the Midwest and the Atlantic and Pacific coasts.

Culturally, the United States is a melting pot of nationalities and traditions, reflected in its music, art, cuisine, and festivities. The influence of diverse communities, including indigenous, African American, Latino, and Asian communities, has enriched American identity.

Economically, it is one of the most significant powers in the world, with a capitalist system that encourages innovation and entrepreneurship. Iconic cities like New York, Los Angeles, and Chicago are commerce, culture, and entertainment centers.

Additionally, the United States is known for its democratic system and role in international politics, being a leader in many areas, from technology to defense. However, they also face challenges like social inequality and the immigration debate. In short, the United States is a country of contrasts and opportunities, where diversity and innovation are a fundamental part of its essence.

W. D. Crano (✉) · E. M. Alvaro · J. T. Siegel
Department of Psychology, Claremont Graduate University, Claremont, CA, USA
e-mail: William.crano@cgu.edu; Eusebio.alvaro@cgu.edu; jason.siegel@cgu.edu

A. Pérez-Gómez, J. Mejía-Trujillo (eds.), *Drug Abuse Prevention*, Advances in Mental Health and Addiction, https://doi.org/10.1007/978-3-031-99621-4_7

Introduction

The history of responses to misuse of substances deemed dangerous in the United States has played a large role in forming public opinion and legal responses for nearly two centuries. Often, psychoactive substance use prevention approaches have been based on little more that guesswork or dogma, relying more on the opinions of their developers than the scientific knowledge of the times. This mistake has been repeated often over the years. Now, with the development of science-based models, there is hope for a more positive response to prevention campaigns, but the strong tendency to revert to less informed approaches is always a danger. In this overview, we trace work on prevention in the United States from beginning to the projected future in terms of governmental plans going forward. Given the magnitude of the task and the many roads that have been taken, this review is of necessity selective, but hopefully it will present a picture of behaviors at times where knowledge was scarce, but opinions plentiful and strongly held.

Beginnings Through—2010

Campaigns to inhibit marijuana uptake were the first formal large-scale psychotropic substance use prevention campaigns in the United States. One of the earliest efforts was launched in the 1880s by the Women's Christian Temperance Union (WCTU: Evans, 2022). The WCTU used fear appeals to advocate abstinence from alcohol, marijuana, and other psychoactive substances. The organization had a strong effect in the country, even resulting in the inclusion of their approach in school textbooks through the 1930s. The end of prohibition (which was fought by the WCTU) and accompanying shifts in public attitudes seriously weakened the organization's influence. Nonetheless, anti-marijuana attitudes persisted in the US government; ultimately marijuana prevention was embraced by the US Federal Bureau of Narcotics in the 1930s where its head, Harry Anslinger, promoted a concerted series of fear-based campaigns, largely unsuccessful, through the late 1950s when he retired (Chasin, 2016).

A New Approach

The early 1960s marked a transition in campaign implementation—taking cues from the WCTU's strategic approach, the US government installed prevention firmly back in schools through coordinated student education. However, this time it was not via formal presentations in dry textbooks but in highly visceral movie shorts shown to a captive student audience in classrooms and school assemblies. The lurid appeals spearheaded by Anslinger were now coupled to the WCTU's educational approach. To paraphrase Marshall McLuhan, while the medium changed the message was resolutely the same—at the core of this effort, fear-based appeals were employed to foster the desired outcome of abstinence. Millions of elementary school students were exposed to countless exaggerated stories of rabid marijuana users throughout the decade to the early 1970s, when the US government released a comprehensive report on the status of substance use in America. The key finding of this report was clear: Scare tactics were not working, and worse, were actually counterproductive (National Commission on Marihuana and Drug Abuse (Farnsworth, 1972, 1973; Nahas & Greenwood, 1973). What followed was a brief abatement of fear-based campaigns with a turn to more reasoned information-based messaging, but few were being implemented. The potential of this approach was not capitalized upon—clearly, information is necessary for enduring change in beliefs (Wood et al., 1995), but it is not sufficient (Crano et al., 2019; Crano et al., 2015), and with the subsequent increasing use of marijuana and other illicit substances in the 1970s, messaging approaches once again reverted to past themes.

Big Media

In the early 1980s, following a change in the US Presidency and new leadership at the National Institute on Drug Abuse (NIDA), prevention campaigns were newly energized around the "Just say no" mantra led by the highly public efforts of First Lady Nancy Reagan. This new guiding message theme was supplemented by the similarly energized use of fear-arousing appeals by the Partnership for a Drug Free America (PDFA). An organization growing out of the sponsorship of tobacco, alcohol, and pharmaceutical companies, the PDFA quickly became a leading source of ensuing prevention campaigns, to the detriment of prevention in the United States.

Established by the Anti-Drug Abuse Act of 1988, the White House Office of National Drug Control Policy (ONDCP) coordinated the United States' drug control efforts. While generally addressing the reduction of illegal substance use distribution-related behaviors (e.g., use, manufacturing, trafficking, etc.), the ONDCP also took an active role in funding and developing mass media substance use prevention campaigns. The next two-plus decades were characterized by large-scale campaigns built on partnerships between the federal government, private industry organizations, and other non-governmental interest groups. Professionally produced messages of a high technical quality would come to typify the new look of substance use prevention campaigns in the United States. Certainly, the look had changed—taking cues, and often with the direct involvement of the advertising industry, the campaigns often took novel, edgy approaches, and eye-catching visuals. While this new model unquestionably assisted in drawing audience attention—addressing a necessary component of successful attitude and behavior change (Crano et al., 2019)—the general persuasion approach of proscribing behavior, yet again largely characterized by fear appeals, failed to build on exposure effects, a necessary but insufficient feature of persuasion-based prevention. In fact, drawing attention to communications featuring misguided message appeals (e.g., fear, exaggeration, etc.) has the potential for iatrogenic effects—further exacerbating the situation (Crano et al., 2015, 2019; Petty & Wegener, 1999; Petty et al., 2013). As will be seen, this danger would become evident in evaluations of subsequent campaigns. Nonetheless, given the renewed interest in substance use prevention via mass media, some promising new message themes managed to emerge. While fear appeals still played a prominent role, in the PDFA's messaging in the 1990s, humor, appeals to social norms, and more novel approaches were now becoming part of the prevention campaign message repertoire.

Arguably the apex of decades of prevention campaigns—at least in terms of campaign expenditures and resultant exposure—was the ONDCP's National Youth Anti-Drug Media Campaign (NYAMC). Active from 1998–2004 under the general "My Anti-Drug" slogan, this approximately $1.4 billion initiative targeted parents, adolescents, and young adults, seeking to empower viewers to develop and strengthen anti-drug attitudes while seeking alternatives to use. While multiple illicit substances were addressed via the campaign, marijuana was a key focus, and adolescents were the key targets. The messaging themes and approaches became more varied—while heavy-handed fear appeals were certainly present, they no longer dominated—especially as the campaign unfolded over the years. However, this welcome change (from the standpoint of effective persuasion) was counteracted by the lack of a coordinated core of theory-based messaging. Instead, aided by large budgets and pro-bono work by creative teams, the ads, although undoubtedly professional-looking and attention-getting, generally featured a plethora of themes that appeared to reflect the whims of campaign "creatives" rather than evidence derived from relevant behavioral science research. Despite consistent branding, campaign momentum failed to materialize owing to the apparent lack of foresight in developing consistent themes and models. While some individual campaign messages were persuasive, they were buried in a sea of other messages that at best were pointless from the standpoint of the adolescent audience, and at worst arousing curiosity about the very substances they were meant to disparage.

The resultant campaign outcomes could be predicted from the apparent randomness of the prevention themes evident in the campaign (Crano et al., 2015): High campaign exposure of poorly designed persuasive communications could only result in overall campaign failure. In fact, extensive campaign evaluation (the most comprehensive to date) revealed iatrogenic effects—increased marijuana use and increased perceptions of usage as normative as correlates of exposure (Ginsburg & Czyzewska, 2005; Hornik et al., 2008). Even worse, these iatrogenic effects were especially pronounced among younger viewers (Scheier & Grenard, 2010). The shame of all of this is that the data of the campaign were reviewed every 6 months, and the lack of effect and possible iatrogenicity were brought to the attention of the campaign managers at ONDCP, but these warnings were minimized or dismissed by those in charge of the campaign. The campaign succeeded in generating some of the highest media campaign exposure ratings ever seen before, but coupled with the disappointing results, proved a point known to many, exceptional message exposure will not overcome exceptionally poor messaging.

The ONDCP was rebranded as “Above the Influence” (ATI), and the campaign was restructured in 2005 to reflect community-based partnerships, with a strong focus on the use of local events and other activities rather than reliance on a monolithic nationwide mass media persuasion campaign. ATI also reflected a shift away from focusing on specific substances to broader concerns believed to underly the initiation of substance use more generally. The new effort endured through 2011, without much impact. Its early findings suggested possible effectiveness, but the program’s takeover by the former ONDCP group effectively ended the program after a promising start. The lack of understanding of how to translate a relatively abstract model—Ajzen’s (1991) theory of planned behavior (TPB)—resulted from a failure to devise a workable and applicable ‘translation’ of the theory, what Merton called a model of the “middle level” in which the abstract factors implicated in TPB were redefied in a way to make them readily usable in applied contexts (Merton, 1968, 1991).

Early Years to the Peak

The earliest decades of substance use prevention campaigns in the United States highlight an interesting ongoing duality—direct involvement of both the government and NGOs (e.g., WCTU). There have been decades where the government has taken the lead, and then relinquished the lead to NGOs that have figured more prominently. Many campaigns can be characterized as national (under the sponsorship of the federal government) of moderately long duration and generally high exposure. This phase culminated in the “My Anti-Drug” campaign, which was active from 1998–2004; the campaign’s massive investment, largely for the purchase of airtime and other paid media to maximize exposure, did little to guarantee its success. The generally acknowledged campaign failure and subsequent turn to more localized outreach and advertising featuring coordination with community organizations would appear to set the stage for a major shift in substance use prevention campaigns in the United States.

2010—Present

Several significant developments occurred in the second decade of the twenty-first century that appear to have had a profound impact on approaches to substance use prevention in the United States. These developments had individual as well as interactive effects. The legalization of marijuana for medical, and then recreational use is directly relevant to efforts directed at the prevention of marijuana use, insofar as the more readily availability of the substance in some states was reflected in a noteworthy increase in adolescent use. Another development—the explosion of social media—had considerably broader societal implications but it too would have a direct impact on substance use prevention campaigns. A new channel—one heavily used by adolescents and young adults—had appeared on the horizon. This presented a considerable challenge to the use of traditional media channels to direct prevention messages to youth, often their primary target audience. This audience had largely deserted mainline media for other outlets that appeared tailored to their interests. These new outlets or channels offered much in the way of opportunity for messaging, audience interaction, and subsequent impact. A third development, with clear origins in the approach taken by ATI in the first decade of the new millennium, was a move away from large coordinated national campaigns to considerably more localized outreach. There was still a role to be played at the national level, but it was more focused on the development of materials that could be used by others in varied communication channels. This new approach, the dominant model to date, features local implementation (and often creation) of materials developed and made available by more centralized organizations.

Substances Addressed

While still illegal at the federal level, in individual states, the decriminalization of marijuana for medical use in various states began in the late 1990s and steadily increased through the 2000s and the 2010s. As of April 2024, 37 of 50 states have passed legislation legalizing the use of marijuana for medical purposes; others have legalized only CBD, which can be synthesized from the marijuana plant. Of the 37 states allowing for medical marijuana, 32 also have "decriminalized" its use. The laws detailing decriminalization vary from state to state in terms of amounts that may be held, grown, etc. (see https://disa.com/marijuana-legality-by-state). The federal government has rated marijuana as a Schedule 1 drug, subject to the same legal sanctions as those levied for use of heroin, but this classification is likely to change in the near term, with a lower scheduled rating assumed.

While prior preventive failures might have raised concerns of those developing and implementing marijuana prevention campaigns, it was the more recent decriminalization of marijuana for recreational use that would introduce more challenges to traditional campaign approaches. Starting in 2012 with the states of Colorado and Washington, the trend toward decriminalization of recreational use in the majority of states in the country has raised the greatest concern. These changes have significant implications for the practical implementation of campaigns as well as the messaging themes likely to be considered and used. On the implementation side, national campaigns proscribing marijuana use became much less feasible due to the differing laws in individual states. More state-specific targeting and tailoring of information is required, even though substance use prevention in the legalized states is still needed. On the messaging side, campaigns focused on youth would now need to contend with the fact that adult use was, in many instances, decriminalized (i.e., legal for all intents and purposes). How then to convince youth that using marijuana is acceptable for adults but not for them? Moreover, what are the implications for how other illicit substances are perceived?

This conundrum also introduced the issue of how to message adults regarding their own use. Thematically, from the start, prevention campaigns often centered on the negative (often-exaggerated), detailing harms of use, general societal disapproval, and vague messages advocating avoidance. While these themes can still be found among more recent efforts—especially when it comes to highlighting emerging substances, there has been an observable shift to address the negative outcomes of use in specific contexts. Responsible use and harm reduction approaches typifying campaigns to mitigate harmful effects of alcohol use would seem to become more relevant and appropriate models of other substance prevention models. Specific contexts would include the use of marijuana while driving, use during pregnancy, and safely securing marijuana to limit availability to children and adolescents. This became a focus in states such as Colorado, Washington, and New York where legislation decriminalized recreational use. Youth access to marijuana purchased by adults in their home also now would become a target.

Focus on New Substances

As history noted, marijuana was one of the earliest substances targeted in the earliest prevention campaigns in the United States and remained a core focus through to the new millennium. Nonetheless, other substances had sporadic appearances in campaigns throughout the decades—cocaine, psychedelics, methamphetamine, heroin, and varied pharmaceuticals were all addressed to some extent at one time or other. In the first decade of the millennium, methamphetamine use, increasing throughout the 1990s, was labeled an epidemic and quickly attracted attention of prevention campaigners. By 2010, a dramatic rise in opioid use and addiction led to similar increased attention from campaign developers. These seemingly more viscerally impactful changes—perhaps especially when coupled with the challenges facing marijuana prevention messaging—led to a strong substance-specific emphasis with some familiar themes from the past. Where many of the existing marijuana prevention messages addressed harm mitigation, campaigns targeting first methamphetamine and then opioids were largely rooted in using threat, fear, and disgust as core message themes. As with similar campaigns from the past, this messaging is far from an ideal persuasive approach (Crano et al., 2015, 2019).

Social Media

The advent and increasing use of the internet through the 1990s and early 2000s led to the adoption of social media as a new communication channel to supplement more traditional media when addressing the prevention of illicit or illegal substances. In some cases, this new channel began to supplant more traditional media forms. Prevention websites propagated, messages appeared as banners on more general sites, and a concurrent decline was seen in the use of television, radio, and print. The emerging medium was significantly cheaper for message placement and had the possibility of increasing exposure via increased viewer time spent on preferred websites (vs. TV/radio ads). More refined targeting and tailoring of prevention messages to desired audiences also was possible in the new medium. Costs were further reduced by the technical features of the medium because content developed for the internet did not need to be broadcast quality. Readily available high quality digital cameras and editing software also greatly reduced production costs.

In the 2010s the expansion and explosive growth of social media, combined with easy access via increasingly ever-present smartphones, threw fuel on already-growing online prevention efforts. The functional feature set of this new technology seemed ready-made for two technical and thematic considerations that had been working through the prevention community in recent decades. On the technical side, proponents of message targeting and tailoring had advocated for the benefits that would obtain from clearly delineating a defined audience and reaching them with a message specifically matched to any number of theoretically proposed variables ranging from biophysiological to social levels. Social media is, by design, eminently amenable to facilitating this view of message dissemination. What of the content of these messages? It turns out that social media also is well-positioned to distribute and amplify message themes that are becoming increasingly popular—most notably messages addressing social norms regarding substance use (Roditis et al., 2016; Wong et al., 2020). Factors central to social media—social networks, content sharing, influencers, etc.—position this communication channel as the central vehicle to promulgate social normative information. Where better to address social norms but within one's social network?

Central Production/Local Dissemination

The change in media formats, from broadcast to digital with ever-increasing interactivity and ever-decreasing cost, is matched by changes in the way substance use prevention campaigns are designed and implemented. Whereas, until now, large scale national programs (e.g., school-based efforts in place from the start) and campaigns were the norm—the NYAMC was the epitome of this phase—the past few decades can be characterized by increased decentralization of implementation and reduced involvement of the federal government. With a few exceptions, for example, Ad Council campaigns addressing the opioid crisis and more recently adolescent vaping, communication efforts are localized (see https://www.adcouncil.org/our-story/our-history). Though the contribution of federal agencies to research and application of prevention of psychoactive substances remains strong, campaigns are more likely to be produced at the state or even county levels, rather than nationally.

Non-governmental efforts also are prominent in more local contexts—even down to individual cities and school districts.

While this change in campaign focus and the resultant reduction in scope has had an impact on campaign development and implementation, perhaps the most dramatic shift can be seen in the production and availability of the content used in current campaigns, and their focus on local issues. While federal support of large-scale campaign implementation appears clearly in decline, various organizations at national level have increasingly become repositories of campaign resources. This clearinghouse model is evident at varied levels of government (county/state/federal) as well as among varied non-governmental organizations also operating from local through national contexts. At the national governmental level, the Substance Use and Mental Health Services Administration (SAMHSA), the National Institute on Drug Abuse (NIDA), and the Drug Enforcement Agency (DEA) among others, all sponsor substance use prevention clearinghouses. National non-governmental actors include Above the Influence/Drugfree.org, Be Under Your Own Influence (2015–2020), Voices for Awareness, National Association of State and Drug Abuse Directors (NASADAD), and many others. The goal of these organizations is to produce a wide variety of content and make it readily accessible and amenable to use across multiple channels at local levels by varied organizations. Perhaps driven by the idea of reaching people where they live, this re-tooling had already begun with the ATI campaign (2005–2011) where the national and highly centralized NYAMC campaign was rebranded and re-configured to provide more localized promotional materials and events.

It is noteworthy that most clearinghouse campaign materials are graphics and slides, which involve low production costs, easy reproducibility, and rapid implementation in physical (i.e., posters, flyers, etc.) and online (i.e., web site and social media banners and posts) applications. Video and audio messages are still available—largely for online use where, as noted, acceptable production value is attainable at low cost.

Where Are We Now?

In all, we now find ourselves in prevention campaign contexts characterized by accessible materials that are implementation-ready across a wide variety of channels, and a concomitant reduction in individual campaign reach and duration. It is arguably a time of great opportunity with equally prominent challenges. The clearinghouse model makes it eminently easy for any interested organization—whether national, regional, or local— to access materials that in their preferred campaign can be implemented at relatively low cost. This greatly facilitates leveraging individuals and contexts more proximate to their targeted audiences, reaching them where they live. The targeting and tailoring potential of this prevention model is apparent. However, given their localized nature, such campaigns usually are shorter, more focused, and often with narrower and less exposure. They lack the considerable resources accruing from the economies of scale possible via national efforts. The resulting concern is whether a sufficiently large prevention "dose" is possible in such systems.

Campaign effectiveness still rests heavily on the nature and quality of the available messages. The messaging to be accessed via a clearinghouse for use in a campaign is entirely dependent on the types of messages produced. Are messages theory- and evidence-based? Are messages pretested? With whom? The wide availability of poor messaging is a recipe for iatrogenic effects or, at minimum, campaign failure. This concern may be further exacerbated by the extent to which materials are customized. How are they being customized? The potential benefits of the best theory- and evidence-based messages can be nullified easily with faulty or whimsical customization, or when presented in the wrong combination. It is evident that education and training in the development of persuasive messages is clearly needed and should be guiding efforts both as to the messages being created for clearinghouses as well as for the end users of those messages.

Going Forward

As will be shown, the trend toward localization of prevention efforts does not indicate a retreat of national funding bodies. For example, the US National Institute on Drug Abuse (NIDA), acting in concert with the ONDCP, is a principal organization in the country in directing drug prevention and treatment. NIDA's funding level for 2024 was $1,663.4 million, 64% of which is spent on extramural grants.[1] Clearly, NIDA's funding priorities and considerable budget have a powerful directive effect on the types and forms of prevention and treatment of psychoactive substance use, but this does not belie the trend toward localization, as many of the projects funded by the organization, while large, are localized, and are supported with diffusion of techniques and results taking on a somewhat less critical feature of funding decisions than the scientific quality of the proffered work. The Institute is focused on the science of prevention, substance initiation, usage, dependence, treatment, recovery, and relapse prevention. Its publicly disseminated plans provide a clear picture of the scope of the Institute, and the broad outlines of these plans are evident in their strategic 5-year plans, the most recent of which was published in late September 2022, when NIDA's governing board released its strategic plan designed to guide the next 5 years of the organization's funding agenda (see https://nida.nih.gov/about-nida/2022-2026-strategic-plan/introduction).

NIDA is the United States' largest funding body for research devoted to the scientific study of psychoactive substance prevention, misuse, and dependence; thus, its strategic plan provides important insights into the agency's priorities related to

[1] See https://nida.nih.gov/about-nida/legislative-activities/budget-information/fiscal-year-2024-budget-information-congressional-justification-national-institute-drug-abuse.

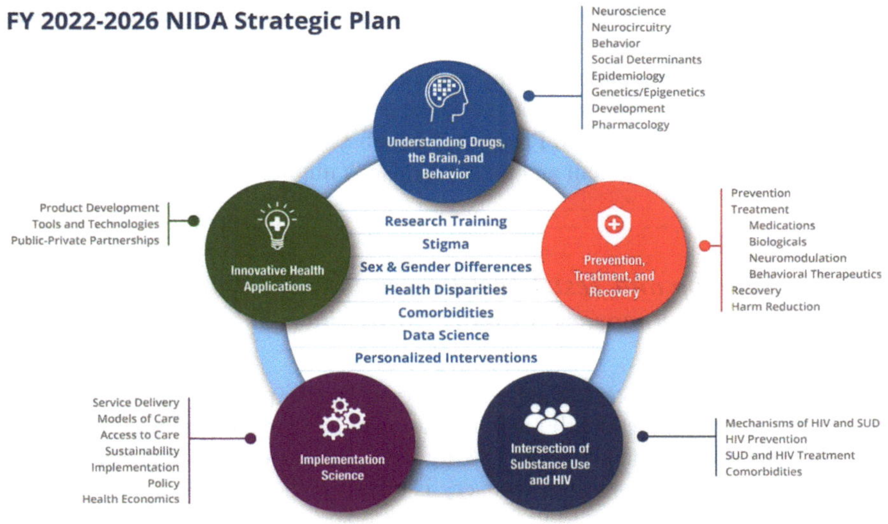

Fig. 1 NIDA Strategic Plan 2022–2026

the control of substance use. NIDA supplies the lion's share of support for all things related to psychoactive substance prevention and treatment in the country.[2] Thus, it is reasonable to inquire into the avenues of this support to understand how it plans to, and likely will impact on the course of prevention and treatment, and the challenges and issues it finds most in need of attention and amelioration in the United States. The old detective novel's cliche, "Follow the money," serves us well in this case.

NIDA's strategic plan is focused on five major goals, or "Priority Scientific Areas," which are understood best via an illustration (Fig. 1).

As indicated in Fig. 1, NIDA funding will be focused on five central goals. They will be considered and discussed in the pages that follow.

Goal 1. Understand Drugs, the Brain, and Behavior

This goal reflects NIDA's basic science orientation, which involves developing deeper understanding of the causes of substance use and addiction. As such, it involves fields of neuroscience, chemistry, medicine, pharmacology, genetics and epigenetics, and behavioral science. The working axiom of the Institute is that addiction is a medical condition, a brain disease. This understanding thus calls for a

[2] Many other organizations (NGOs, religious organizations, etc.) work in more limited ways throughout the country, but NIDA, as the largest funder in the nation, sets the agenda and dictates much of the future of substance use prevention and treatment in the United States.

focus on the brain and the impact of psychotropic substances on the brain. Studies of gene-environment interactions, neural circuitry affected in substance use and addiction, and a greater understanding of the contexts amenable to substance uptake, users and their worlds, methods of substance consumption, and other social factors also are a part of the first goal. Prevention of substance uptake, facilitating maintenance of successful treatment and recovery, also is implicated in this goal.

Goal 2. Develop and Test Novel Prevention, Treatment, Harm Reduction, and Recovery Support Strategies

NIDA's second goal is concerned with interventions to prevent initiation of risky substances or reduce the likelihood of new users moving into the more serious phase of substance use disorders (SUD). The urgency of the issue of primary prevention, harm reduction, and supporting recovery is clearly indicated, given the incredible rate of increasing death due to various psychotropic substances which seem all too readily available (see Fig. 2). Clearly, the usage rates of dangerous substances and

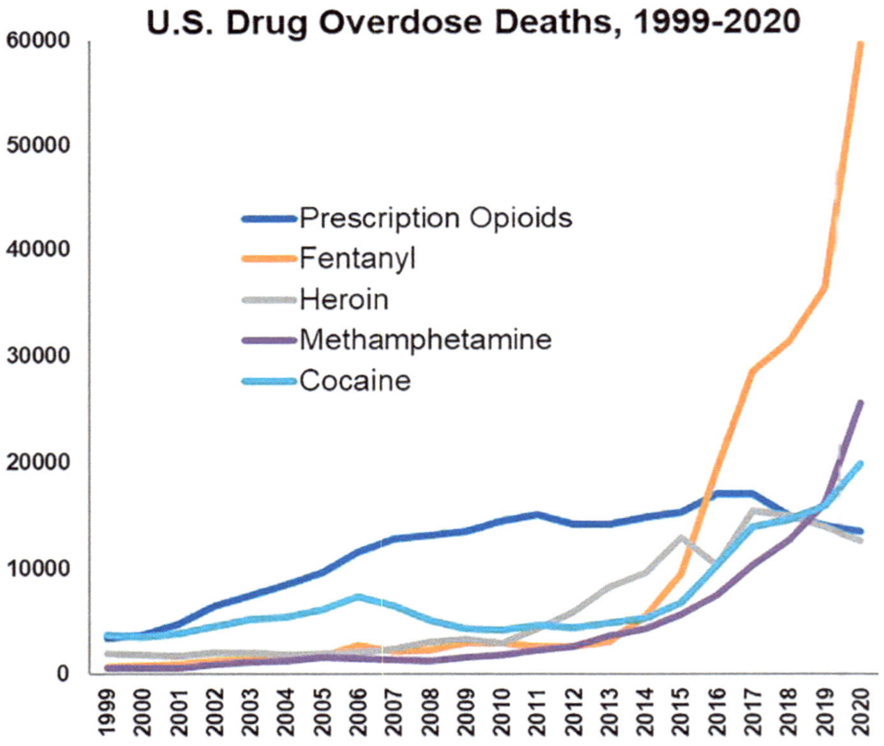

Fig. 2 Overdose deaths in the United States over the past 20 years

their accompanying morbidity and mortality rates are intolerable, and this explains the palpable urgency of Goal 2 as a priority scientific goal. The goal stresses not only the feasibility of prevention models, but also their cost effectiveness. Most would argue that considering costs in lost lives and lost contributions to society, the benefit-to-cost ratio of successful prevention models would almost certainly prove massively positive. This goal calls for new strategies, and this is reasonable as many earlier ones have failed. It also speaks to the need to accelerate research on harm reduction. Research has lagged in this area, as has research on useful techniques that deal with recovery support.

Note the incredible rise in deaths attributed to Fentanyl, Methamphetamines, Cocaine, whereas death attributable to heroin and misuse of prescription opioids have gradually tapered off from 2016–2020.

Goal 3. Accelerate Research on the Intersection of Substance Use, HIV, and Related Comorbidities

The third of NIDA's high priority scientific goals is concerned with the relation between psychoactive substance use and HIV (and other related comorbidities, like Hepatitis). There appears a relation between these two hazards, for two reasons, but the relation is not established as well as it should. The first is that use of substances may interfere with pharmaceuticals that help control progression of HIV into AIDS. The second hazard is that intoxication by alcohol or other psychoactive substances can result in a relaxation of caution which might lead to risky behaviors that otherwise might be avoided. This is a worthy goal, as the relation between substance use and HIV infection is not as well established as might be hoped.

Considering the somewhat unsettled state of knowledge in the area, this third goal has three subsequent actions of high priority. The first is gaining a better understanding of the development, spread, and persistence of HIV infections in the drug-using community. The second is to mitigate new infections and the spread of HIV among drug users and their partners. The third major subgoal is to alleviate comorbidities of those with HIV who also use psychoactive substances.

Goal 4. Improve the Implementation of Evidence-Based Strategies in Real-World Settings

The fourth high priority scientific goal involves the application of evidence-based prevention science to psychoactive substance use prevention and treatment in the field. Generalization of scientifically based research results is never guaranteed (Crano et al., 2024), but the necessity to move laboratory-based findings to the field and to evaluate their success rigorously is practically nonnegotiable considering current rates of morbidity and mortality attributed to substance misuse. There has been a literal explosion of death due to fentanyl overdose in the United States, which has caused massive concern in user and non-user communities. For example, the Centers for Disease Control and Health (CDC) reported a five-fold increase in Fentanyl deaths in the United States from 2016 to 2021 (Spencer et al., 2023), and the national (US) overall death rate is 21.6 deaths per 100,000 residents; death rates are up 30% year-over-year (National Center for Drug Use Statistics, nd: https://drugabusestatistics.org/drug-overdose-deaths/). Translating the dry percentages into whole numbers provides a clearer picture of the toll that one substance, misused on a single occasion, can wreak on an individual, but it does not indicate the effects on their friends and families.

In responding to these astounding and calamitous results, NIDA has wisely prescribed more rapid movement of applications of hard-won basic research knowledge to applied settings in which their need is clear. The transfer of knowledge from laboratory to field applications is never easy, and when the transfer involves prevention in high-risk groups or treatment in substance-use dependent groups, the mere mechanics of amelioration can be daunting. Nevertheless, the payoffs can be great. For example, the World Health Organization (WHO) estimated that every dollar spent in school-based primary prevention in the United States would return approximately $18 in savings. Across the 50 states, this translates to $1.3 billion savings in state and local government spending, and a reduction of approximately a $33.5 billion reduction in lifetime societal costs of medical expenditures and lost productivity nationwide (WHO, 2000). Likewise, implementation of evidence-based treatment models can reduce demand and provide great returns on investment. Research by the International Narcotics Control Board (INCB: 2011) showed that every dollar spent on treatment resulted in a saving of $4–12 in reduced health care and crime costs (International Narcotics Control Board, 2011). Despite these well-founded estimates by some of the world's leading organizations in the service of substance use prevention and treatment, the fact is undeniable that the funding needed to approach a fair chance of obtaining a positive outcome is woefully inadequate. As long as this fact remains true, it is unrealistic to assume that current trends in uptake of dangerous substance will moderate.

Goal 5. Translate Research into Innovative Health Applications

NIDA's fifth priority scientific area is concerned with research utilization for risky psychoactive substance use prevention. This goal is facilitated through two substance-prevention goals, the first of which involves facilitating research translation via education and industry partnerships, and the second, which involves capitalizing new techniques to deliver interventions fostering prevention, treatment, and recovery from substance use. This model follows two programs that have been in effect in many of the agencies of the National Institutes of Health, including NIDA. The Small Business Innovation Research (SBIR) grants and the Small

Business Technology Transfer (SBTT) grants, both of which are designed to integrate academic researchers with individuals and small entrepreneurial enterprises to bring the fruits of scientific research to American society. The SBIR is perhaps the more "academic" and speculative of the two, as its purpose is to join researchers' innovators and their research products with entrepreneurs who can develop business applications that might enrich the lives of the citizenry (and the principals involved in the research and dissemination). The unique feature of this marriage of academe and business is that the profits that accrue to the project are owned by the team, not the government. The same system is in place for the SBTT grants, which takes science-based technological innovations and seeks to disseminate them in commercial form, again for the benefit of the citizenry, with the profits of successful tech transfers accruing to the partners in the enterprise, not the government. This technology transfer program is a common feature of many corporate business operations, but is rare in governmental contexts. It is important to note, that the SBIR and SBTT programs are not small. As shown in their website, NIDA's promotion of these programs and the importance to its mission, cannot be mistaken:

Each year, NIDA provides more than $50 million in awards to small businesses through the Small Business programs. **That's up to $3.4 million in funding per project and all equity remains with grantees** (https://nida.nih.gov/funding/small-business-innovation-research-sbir-technology-transfer-sttr-programs).

With a commitment of $50 million in 2024, it is obvious these programs are considered highly important for the welfare of the country, and they have produced important innovations in substance prevention and treatment. For a description of some of these innovations, see: (https://archives.nida.nih.gov/news-events/noras-blog/2019/10/nidas-help-startups-translate-addiction-science-new-technologies). Eligibility for these programs involve varying proportions of US ownership, company size (less than 500) employees, and other factors. For more information on eligibility see (https://nida.nih.gov/funding/small-business-innovation-research-sbir-technology-transfer-sttr-programs/about-sbir-sttr-programs/program-eligibility).

Past and Future

The NIDA 5-year plan provides a useful and largely accurate picture of the likely future of persuasive research support on substance use prevention available at the federal level. The plan is flexible, it is not a set of ironclad rules designed to dictate course of research, and it is backed by the millions of research dollars made available by the Institute. The program offers a way that a large cadre of dedicated professionals who are at work on prevention of risky substances, within and outside of government service, to indicate their best judgment about the likely needs of the country going forward. If these needs change—e.g., a rapid and unacceptable rate of deaths from a new substance— the organization is flexible enough to direct funds to help alleviate or attenuate the unanticipated problem. With the continuing movement in the United States to a balkanization of the prevention arena, it is reasonable to consider the likelihood that the day of Big Prevention—large scale mass media campaigns, centrally organized and funded— may have come to an end, and grants funded by the Institute may follow the trend to support projects devoted more to local than national issues, unless circumstances require a change in the pendulum's arc to solving issues affecting the country as a whole. Obviously, accurately predicting the future developmental trends of a dynamic area like substance use and prevention is never guaranteed, but the flexibility evinced by NIDA suggests that the adroitness exhibited in the past when changes of direction were indicated will serve the United States, and prevention in general, well in the coming years. We believe the future of substance misuse prevention in the United States is improving. We have learned much about how to deal with issues as they arise, and even how to anticipate those whose problems are likely to fade without intervention, but this assumes we are capable of learning from past mistakes. Of course, this capability is never guaranteed.

Some Concluding Remarks

The current chapter offers a selective discussion of broad-based trends in prevention, starting with some of the earliest attempts, which were alive and well in the late 1800s. As shown throughout, the pendulum of interest and investment has swung from large, nationalized projects to more local approaches, and back again to large scale national efforts. Today, the pendulum seems to have swung again toward localized efforts aided and abetted by federal funding agencies, a combination that promise to enrich both theory and application. This progression is neither good nor bad; rather it characterizes the reality of prevention in the United States. The success or failure of the anticipated localized approaches requires adoption prevention practices that take advantage of scientific evidence. Although it is wildly overused today, the term "evidence based" is both valuable and proper. If we follow established scientific findings properly translated into practice, the future is bright. If this approach is rejected in favor of hubris, whim, or appeals to "common sense," an all too rare commodity, the uneven path of success found over the past 150 years will be replicated. With the ever-growing power of psychoactive substances to cause mortal harm, their relative availability and low cost, it is not likely that we have another century or so to come to grips with the issue of effective prevention. Too often, politics rather than science have guided efforts. Parents and politicians might cheer messages that exaggerate harm and attempt to frighten youth into drug abstinence. These messages might be gratifying and allow decision-makers to feel they are doing God's work, but the sad fact is that such tactics often cause more harm than good. All too often, failure to adopt established principles of communication and persuasion characterize our preventive efforts. Most of these could have been avoided by better training in message construction and more sober understanding of the role of proper methods of prevention, many of which involve developing communications that were guided by established principles of persuasion.

Something Is Not Always Better Than Nothing

Substance prevention methods (e.g., mass media campaigns, PSAs, homemade video spots and blogs, Instagram messages, etc.) that are not based on strong and validated approaches are as likely to fail or cause harm as they are to succeed. There are a host of examples of well-intended pro-social messages failing to influence the usage behaviors they sought to curtail, or in the worst case, encouraging their further use. There is a reason why tobacco companies rarely use explicit and controlling language to court potential smokers into the fold. They are likely aware of frameworks such as psychological reactance theory (Brehm, 1966; see Rosenberg & Siegel, 2017 for a review), which explain that messages threatening the autonomy of message recipients are likely to backfire. There are many examples, in numerous contexts, of well-intended messages backfiring. Well-intended messages have caused vaccination rates to decrease (Sato & Takasaki, 2021), undesirable energy consumption (Schultz et al., 2007), an increase in the desire to smoke (Hyland & Birrell, 1979), and increased favorable attitudes toward violence (Cárdaba et al., 2016). Developers of substance prevention approaches must take such outcomes to heart and create methods that respect the freedom of its recipients to choose while strategically guiding potential and current users away from harmful decisions.

Prevention Audiences Are Not Blank Slates

As described in this review, decades of substance preventive messaging have exaggerated the harms associated with marijuana use. Adults currently in their 50s grew up being told to "just say no" and that their brains would be akin to an egg in a frying pan if they used marijuana. Young adults in their 20s and 30s likely recall being told that marijuana use funded terrorism. In the current environment where marijuana is largely legalized in the United States and many of the threatened outcomes have not come to pass, it is likely that most adults do not trust, and worse yet, perceive little value from most substance-preventive models. This is cause for some degree of pessimism, because if an audience has resisted or demeaned many past prevention efforts, their certainty of their established position grows, and with successive resistance experiences continues to grow, ultimately resulting beliefs and behaviors that can be exceptionally difficult to change (Briñol et al., 2004; Tormala et al., 2006; Tormala & Rucker 2022). Moreover, later unsuccessful prevention efforts will further confirm the belief that anti-drug messages have no value, leading to an even more significant negative bias when the next preventive communication is encountered. This cycle can have a powerful influence, reinforcing parents' and adolescents' mistrust of substance use prevention communications. The negative bias developed from the exaggerations of past campaigns cannot be ignored. This is particularly unfortunate as drugs currently available, such as fentanyl, oxycontin, and the like, indeed have the devastating outcomes that were falsely promised in earlier marijuana prevention efforts. Fortunately, the current expectations are not a death sentence for future campaigns and can work in favor of today's new prevention models.

Theory Must Guide Prevention Approaches

Theories amenable to prevention are widespread and useful. Ajzen's theory of planned behavior, Brehm's (1966) psychological reactance theory, Lasswell's (1948, 1951) two-step flow of communication, Petty et al.' (2013) elaboration likelihood model, and Hovland and collaborators' (1953) message-learning model have all been widely examined in field and laboratory, and all rank as major theoretical frameworks among the myriad theoretical advancements in psychological science over the past century. Their application, when done properly, has been met with considerable success. The challenge is "translating" the abstractions of theory to practice. This translation often is difficult but far from impossible, and the proper use of well-realized theory in wide-scale or even modest campaigns can address important issues effectively across diverse audiences. Fentanyl might be a relatively new drug, but substance prevention campaign developers are not starting from scratch when developing the best ways of preventing and reducing its use. We implore campaign developers to take advantage of the decades upon decades of research on persuasion and prevention science and allow the lessons of the past to guide future approaches. As described, a "spray and leave" approach to messaging is a poor use of resources, and over the years has caused considerable harm.

Extensive Pilot Testing Is Indispensable and Non-negotiable

About a decade ago, the authors of this chapter conducted focus groups with adolescents. We showed the adolescents six anti-marijuana messages that had been used in a multi-million-dollar prevention campaign conducted in the United States over 4 years. The outcome of the campaign was a disaster. From the initiation of the massive program, our opinion of the campaign communications was that they were unlikely to involve or impress the assembled nationally representative audience of adolescent students, 12 to 18 years of age, the focal target of the campaign. Our evaluation indicated that initially abstinent students who rejected some of the most popular campaign communications were significantly more likely than those who evaluated the messages positively to initiate marijuana use in the following year (Alvaro et al., 2013). This finding indicates that danger lies ahead for young adolescents who reject substance-preventive communications. The rejection of the preventive material rendered them more susceptible to later inducements to use the proscribed substance. We do not know if the expensive campaign's messages were pilot tested prior to implementation, but in our research, adolescents' responses made it clear that more extensive preliminary message testing was needed. It is foolish to go into the field with an expensive persuasion campaign if the messages' comprehensibility and persuasiveness have not been established in prior preliminary research—and almost all prevention campaigns are expensive, if not in financial terms, then in terms of potentially lost opportunities.

A Final Note

It is clearly in the best interest of society for adolescents to abstain from imbibing alcohol, smoking cigarettes, or smoking/vaping/consuming marijuana, common "starter" drugs for most adolescents in the United States who do not remain abstinent. None of these substances facilitate good health or proper cognitive development. Many prevention campaigns launched with high hopes and the best intentions have failed to deliver on our promise to youth to do our best for them. Some campaigns, even multi-million-dollar campaigns, have increased the likelihood that some adolescents will adopt marijuana use, whereas if the campaign went unnoticed, they would not have done so (see Hornik et al., 2008). This is disturbing in many different ways. If the same missteps are made with drugs like Fentanyl, many will likely die as a result. The drugs of today are too dangerous for politics and amateurs to design and implement persuasive preventive approaches. Campaign developers must learn from the successes and failures of the past and allow science alone to guide future efforts.

References

Ajzen, I. (1991). The theory of planned behavior. *Organizational Behavior and Human Decision Processes*, *50*(2), 179-211. https://doi.org/10.1016/0749-5978(91)90020-t (Theories of cognitive self-regulation)

Alvaro, E. M., Crano, W. D., Siegel, J. T., Hohman, Z., Johnson, I., & Nakawaki, B. (2013). NSPY Ad evaluation, marijuana use status, and future marijuana use. *Psychology of Addictive Behaviors*. https://doi.org/10.1037/a0031960

Brehm, J. W. (1966). A theory of psychological reactance. Academic Press.

Briñol, P., Rucker, D. D., Tormala, Z. L., & Petty, R. E. (2004). Individual differences in resistance to persuasion: The role of beliefs and meta-beliefs. In E. S. Knowles & J. A. Linn (Eds.), Resistance and persuasion. (pp. 83–104). Lawrence Erlbaum Associates Publishers.

Cárdaba, M. A. M., Briñol, P., Brändle, G., & Ruiz-San Román, J. A. (2016). The moderating role of aggressiveness in response to campaigns and interventions promoting anti-violence attitudes. *Aggressive Behavior, 42*(5), 471–482.

Chasin, A. (2016). Asasin of youth; A kaleidoscopic history of Harry J. Ansinger's War on Drugs. University of Chicago Press.

Crano, W. D., Alvaro, A. M., & Siegel, J. T. (2019). Creative persuasive substance-use prevention communications: The EQUIP model. In Z. Sloboda, H. Petras, E. Robertson, & R. W. Hingson (Eds.), *Prevention of substance use* (pp. 303-318). Springer Nature Switzerland.

Crano, W. D., Alvaro, E. M., & Siegel, J. T. (2015). The media campaign as a focal prevention strategy: A guide to design, implementation, and evaluation. In L. M. Scheier (Ed.), *Handbook of adolescent drug use prevention: Research, intervention strategies, and practice* (pp. 397-414). American Psychological Association. https://doi.org/10.1037/14550-023

Crano, W. D., Brewer, M. B., & Lac, A. (2024). *Principles and methods of social research* (4 ed.). Routledge.

Evans, C. H. (2022). Do everything: The biography of Frances Willard. Oxford Univerity Press.

Farnsworth, D. L. (1972). Summary of the report from the National Commission on Marihuana and Drug Abuse: Marihuana: A signal of misunderstanding. *Psychiatric Annals*, *2*(5), 8-25. https://doi.org/10.3928/0048-5713-19720501-04

Farnsworth, D. L. (1973). The second report of the National Commission on Marihuana and Drug Abuse: Background and recommendations. *Psychiatric Annals*, *3*(4), 14-47. https://doi.org/10.3928/0048-5713-19730401-04

Ginsburg, H. J. & Czyzewska, M. (2005). "National anti-marijuana ads compared to anti-tobacco ads: differences between immediate favorable and unfavorable post-viewing written comments." North American Journal of Psychology **7**(3).

Hornik, R. C., Jacobsohn, L., Orwin, R., Piesse, A., & Kalton, G. (2008). Effects of the National Youth Anti-drug Media Campaign on youths. *American Journal of Public Health*, *98*, 2229-2236.

Hovland, C. I., Janis, I. L., & Kelley, H. H. (1953). *Communication and persuasion: Psychological studies of opinion change*. Yale University Press. http://search.ebscohost.com/login.aspx?direct=true&db=psyh&AN=1964-00891-000&site=ehost-live

Hyland, M., & Birrell, J. (1979). Government health warnings and the boomerang effect. *Psychological Reports, 44*(2), 643–647. https://doi.org/10.2466/pr0.1979.44.2.643

InternationalNarcoticsControlBoard. (2011). Annual Report. Retrieved May 24 2019, from https//www.incg.org/documents/Publications/AnnualReport/Thematic_Chapters/English/AR_2013_E_Chapter_1.pdf

Lasswell, H. D. (1948). The structure and function of communication in society. In L. Bryson (Ed.), *The communication of ideas: A series of addresses* (pp. 37-51). Institute for Religious and Social Studies.

Lasswell, H. D. (1951). *Political writings of Harold D. Lasswell*. Free Press.

Merton, R. K. (1968). *Social Theory and Social Structure (1968 enlarged ed.)*. Free Press.

Merton, R. K. (1991). *Introduction to sociology*. Harcourt Brace Jovonovich.

Nahas, G., & Greenwood, A. (1973). A critique of the first report of the National Commission on Marihuana and Drug Abuse (1972). *Psychiatric Annals*, *3*(4), 94-106. https://doi.org/10.3928/0048-5713-19730401-07

NIDA. 2022a, October 19. Director's Message. Retrieved from https://nida.nih.gov/about-nida/2022-2026-strategic-plan/directors-message on 2022, retrieved October 12, 2020.

NIDA. 2022b, September 21. NIDA Releases Its 2022-2026 Strategic Plan. Retrieved from https://nida.nih.gov/about-nida/noras-blog/2022/09/nida-releases-its-2022-2026-strategic-plan on 2022. Retrieved October 15, 2022

Petty, R. E., & Wegener, D. T. (1999). The elaboration likelihood model: Current status and controversies. In S. Chaiken & Y. Trope (Eds.), *Dual-process theories in social psychology.* (pp. 37-72). Guilford Press. http://search.ebscohost.com/login.aspx?direct=true&db=psyh&AN=1999-02377-002&site=ehost-live

Petty, R. E., Wheeler, S. C., & Tormala, Z. L. (2013). Persuasion and attitude change. In H. Tennen, J. Suls, & I. B. Weiner (Eds.), *Handbook of psychology, Vol. 5: Personality and social psychology (2nd ed.).* (pp. 369-389). John Wiley & Sons Inc. http://search.ebscohost.com/login.aspx?direct=true&db=psyh&AN=2012-28461-017&site=ehost-live&scope=site

Roditis, M. L., Delucchi, K., Chang, A., & Halpern-Felsher, B. (2016). Perceptions of social norms and exposure to pro-marijuana messages are associated with adolescent marijuana use. *Preventive Medicine: An International Journal Devoted to Practice and Theory*, *93*, 171-176. https://doi.org/10.1016/j.ypmed.2016.10.013

Rosenberg, B. D., & Siegel, J. T. (2017). A 50-Year Review of Psychological Reactance Theory: Do Not Read This Article. Motivation Science. https://doi.org/10.1037/mot0000091

Scheier, L. M., & Grenard, J. L. (2010). Influence of a nationwide social marketing campaign on adolescent drug use. *Journal of Health Communication, 15, I240-271.*

Sato, R., & Takasaki, Y. (2021). Vaccine hesitancy and refusal: behavioral evidence from rural northern Nigeria. *Vaccines, 9*(9), 1023. https://doi.org/10.3390/vaccines9091023

Schultz, P. W., Nolan, J. M., Cialdini, R. B., Goldstein, N. J., & Griskevicius, V. (2007). The constructive, destructive, and reconstructive power of social norms. *Psychological Science, 18*(5), 429–434.

Spencer, M. R., Warner, M., Cisewski, J. A., Minino, A., Dodds, D., Perera, J., & Ahmad, F. B. (2023). Estimates of drug overdose deaths involving Fentanyl, Methamphetamine, Cocaine, Heroin, and Oycodone: United States, 2021. *NVSS: Vital Statistics Rapid Release, Report No. 27.* https://www.cdc.gov/nchs/data/vsrr/vsrr027.pdf

Tormala, Z. L., Clarkson, J. J., & Petty, R. E. (2006). Resisting persuasion by the skin of one's teeth: The hidden success of resisted persuasive messages. *Journal of Personality and Social Psychology, 91*(3), 423–435. https://doi.org/10.1037/0022-3514.91.3.423

Tormala, Z. L., & Rucker, D. D. (2022). Attitude change and persuasion: Classic, metacognitive, and advocacy perspectives. In APA handbook of consumer psychology. (pp. 323–350). American Psychological Association. https://doi.org/10.1037/0000262-013

WHO. (2000). Primary prevention of substance abuse: A workbook for project operators. Retrieved 10 December 2022, from https://www.unodc.org/pdf/globalinitiative/initiative_activities_workbook.pdf

Wong, S.-W., Buu, A., & Lin, H.-C. (2020). State medical marijuana laws and associated marijuana use, attitudes, and perceived social norms among adolescents in the US. *Journal of Psychoactive Drugs, 52*(5), 383-392. https://doi.org/10.1080/02791072.2020.1795325

Wood, W., Rhodes, N., & Biek, M. (1995). Working knowledge and attitude strength; An informational processing analysis. In R. E. Petty & J. A. Krosnick (Eds.), *Attitude strength: Antecedents and consequences*. Psychology Press.

William D. Crano is the Oskamp Distinguished Professor of Psychology at Claremont Graduate University. His research focuses on persuasion and self-interest on attitudes and actions. His current work deals with developing persuasive methods to prevent substance use in adolescents and young adults. Crano was a NATO Senior Scientist, a Fulbright Fellow, a liaison scientist in the US Office of Naval Research (London), and director of the Program in Social Psychology at the National Science Foundation.

Eusebio M. Alvaro is a Professor of Psychology and Associate Provost for Research at Claremont Graduate University. His basic research is on social influence processes such as biased message processing, resistance to persuasion, indirect message effects, and minority influence. He conducts applied persuasion for health promotion/disease prevention focusing on developing and testing media communications. Key-funded research includes substance use prevention, organ donation, diabetes prevention, and community mental health.

Jason T. Siegel is a Professor of Psychology at Claremont Graduate University, where he directs the Depression and Persuasion Research Lab and co-directs the Health Psychology and Prevention Science Institute. Dr. Siegel applies theories of persuasion and motivation to create messages for increasing help-seeking among people with depression, reducing the stigmatization of people with depression, increasing organ donor registration behavior, and reducing substance abuse in adolescents.

Pilot Implementation of an Intervention in Life Skills with Argentine and Brazilian Youth: Challenges and Potential in the Prevention of Drug Use in an Educational Context

María Elena Iturriaga Goroso, Thaís Soares Pereira, and Telmo Mota Ronzani

Mental Health Problems Among Adolescents

According to the Pan American Health Organization (PAHO, 2017), the adolescent and young population represents 30% of Latin America and the Caribbean; however, at the same time that the population will continue to increase in the coming decades, mortality rates are increasing, with adolescent suicide being one of the main causes (Economic Commission for Latin America [ECLAC], 2022; PAHO, 2017).

The prevalence of mental disorders in adolescents shows that in Latin America children between 10 and 14 years old present 7% while those between 15 and 19 years old present 8%; observing that anxiety and depression represent 50% of mental health problems in the population between 10 and 19 years old (Pan-American Life, 2022). Likewise, occupying second place in chronic non-communicable diseases are mental, neurological disorders and the use of psychoactive substances, which are responsible for 20% of the burden of morbidity, disability, premature death, increasing the risk of other health problems (Pan-American Life, 2022). According to PAHO results (2017), there are inequalities in access to treatment for mental disorders, being 82.2% in children and adolescents.

Particularly, in Argentina, based on the report carried out by the United Nations Children's Fund [UNICEF] (2021) about the emotions and impact on mental health

This chapter is the result of the project "Life skills and prevention of substance use in a school context: psychosocial intervention with young people in social vulnerability", funded by Fundação de Amparo à Pesquisa de Minas Gerais (FAPEMIG), process number APQ-03190- 22.

M. E. I. Goroso · T. S. Pereira · T. M. Ronzani (✉)
Department of Psychology, Universidade Federal de Juiz de Fora (UFJF), Juiz de Fora, Brazil

A. Pérez-Gómez, J. Mejía-Trujillo (eds.), *Drug Abuse Prevention*, Advances in Mental Health and Addiction, https://doi.org/10.1007/978-3-031-99621-4_8

of the pandemic in adolescents between 13 and 18 years old, it is concluded that between August 2020 and February 2021, 66% of adolescents presented anguish and sadness compared to 50% in the last measurement, thus they also expressed feeling loneliness in 31%, subsequently increasing to 32%; likewise, a reduction in irritability was observed from 68% in the first measurement to 49%, and reluctance and/or withdrawal from 52% to 39%. On the contrary, changes in diet and sleep were maintained at 54%. Regarding the feeling of sadness, it was more frequent among adolescents. In this period, 18% of adolescents consulted with a professional for a mental health problem. Such a professional corresponded to a general practitioner in 57%, a psychologist in 56%, and a nurse in 21%. Another relevant data refers to the fact that 14% of adolescents wanted to make a consultation, but could not. In turn, regarding the perception of adolescents between 13 and 18 years old, about a more violent environment during the pandemic, it was 23%, while in the first measurement it was 19%, which increased compared to the pre-pandemic. Although in the last evaluation the feelings of anguish, loneliness, irritability, listlessness, and sadness decreased, it was observed that they triggered a mental health problem, with the majority of respondents stating that they knew friends who experimented in a higher percentage with alcohol and other drugs (UNICEF, 2021).

Data from adolescents in Brazil show that 1 in 6 of them between 10 and 19 years old lives with a mental disorder (UNICEF, 2022). It is highlighted that during the pandemic, 35% felt anxiety while 11% were worried about themselves and 9% and 8% reported feeling indifferent and depressed (UNICEF, 2022). 50% of young people maintained that they felt the need to ask for help, however, 40% did not do so for various reasons such as fear of being judged, insecurity, or lack of knowledge of places of care. Of those who sought help, 20% turned to friends, 15% to psychologists or psychiatrists, 11% to family, 8% to their partner; and finally 2% to teachers and another 2% to professionals of the single health system (SUS) (UNICEF, 2022). Furthermore, the Brazilian Institute of Geography and Statistics (IBGE) in its 2021 report states that, in adolescents between 13 and 17 years old, 63.3% have already used alcohol, and that 34.6% experimented with said drug. Before the age of 14, 13% used some illicit drug such as cocaine, ecstasy, crack, and marijuana. Regarding early initiation of such consumption, adolescent girls present a higher risk of 36.8% compared to adolescents of 32.3%. 15.7% expressed that the use of such substances had consequences such as conflicts in family, friends, and school. These results were obtained before the pandemic and it is inferred that they could have worsened during the post-pandemic (IBGE, 2021).

It is essential to emphasize that the social determinants of mental health influence the suffering of young people, such as living conditions, socioeconomic problems, situations of social exclusion, difficulty in accessing basic services and social support (World Health Organization). Health [WHO], 2021). Therefore, it is essential to generate protective environments in different environments such as the family, school, and the community in general, in order to provide modalities for coping with stressful situations, constituting the development of skills to cultivate healthy interpersonal relationships as one of strategies to promote well-being, among others also related to physical care (WHO, 2021). In this way, the UNICEF study (2021) states that according to the socioeconomic level of Argentine adolescents, the pandemic meant the opportunity for reflection and enjoyment of leisure, while for those from low-middle socioeconomic strata it implied boredom, as well as ambivalent feelings. Among the factors that can contribute to psychosocial suffering are those related to not feeling understood and distancing from significant adults, whether family members or school teachers, and, therefore, the fragility of social ties. Aspects linked to violence in different contexts, such as those linked to housing and economic deficiencies, also exert a certain influence on such problems.

Development of Health Promoting Actions in Schools

Regarding the approach to health in school contexts, certain policies have been carried out in Argentina with the aim of promoting the health-promoting role of institutions, highlighting a comprehensive, participatory, and intersectoral work perspective. From the Pan American Health Organization and the World Health Organization (PAHO & WHO, 2018), the guidelines of the Health Promoting Schools Strategy (EPS) were proposed, which tends to plan and develop continuous actions over time to generate healthy physical and psychosocial environments for all members of the educational community. Therefore, it is concerned with promoting the development of certain competencies, the same being cognitive, emotional, and social in order to enable decision-making about one's own health and that of the community in which the subject lives (PAHO & WHO, 2018). Thus, this strategy seeks to improve the quality of life of students, teachers, and other members by creating a healthy environment that, together with policies at a micro and macrosocial level, influence the guidelines for promoting health. Therefore, the school is not only defined by its role in the teaching-learning process but also by its potential to contribute to the integral development of subjects through the transformation of their environments. The role of the educational institution therefore lies in educating in health, since health is built in its daily social relationships, influencing the risk or protective behaviors of young people and adults who belong to said institution. Work in the psychosocial environment, particularly, contributes through participation and interpersonal relationships between members and families, to adequately resolve conflicts, offering greater emotional well-being. It is here that, among other objectives pursued, observe the importance of deepening and promoting the acquisition of life skills to educate about health in schools (PAHO & WHO, 2018).

Recently in Argentina, the Ministry of Health of the Nation (2021) approved resolution 2198/2021 which deals with the initiative of the National Healthy Environments Strategy, which promotes "a culture of healthy habits and modify the lifestyles of the educational community, thus improving the quality of life and psychosocial health in general and increasing the life expectancy of the population involved" (Ministry of Health, 2021). The goals that are proposed to be achieved refer to institutional strengthening policies in addition to preventing and intervening on the risk factors of non-communicable diseases; as well as promote personal well-being and strengthen healthy interpersonal ties with a human rights perspective (Ministry of Health, 2021). For its part, in 2013, National Law 26,892 emerged on the "Promotion of coexistence and addressing social conflict in educational institutions," which aims to regulate the social life of institutions, prevent violence and harassment through social networks, as well as promote respect for others and the culture of peace (Ministry of Education, 2018). Likewise, there are other regulations that deal with the promotion of supportive coexistence and respect for others, guaranteeing the exercise of the rights of children and adolescents, such as the National Education Law 26.206/06 and the National Law for the Comprehensive Protection of Children's Rights, Boys, Girls, and Adolescents No. 26,061/05 (Ministry of Education, 2018). Within this approach, one of the proposals to achieve a healthy coexistence in schools prioritizing the rights and guarantees of children and adolescents, young people and adults; deals with Life Skills (HpV) in accordance with the guidelines of the World Health Organization.

On the other hand, the official documents that guide Brazilian education, including the National Curricular Parameters (Ministry of Education of Brazil [MEC], 1997) and the Common National Curriculum Base (MEC, 2018), although they do not specifically refer to the concept of Life Skills proposed by the WHO, the need to promote competencies related to said concept among students is presented. With the aim of providing training based on ethical parameters and with emphasis on cognitive, physical, emotional, social and interpersonal aspects, the role of the school as a promoter of essential skills for the comprehensive training of subjects is highlighted (MEC, 1997). In this area, the incentive to self-knowledge, the recognition and management of one's own emotions and those of others is highlighted as the responsibility of basic education; the development of critical and creative thinking; valuing the resolution of problems associated with the various areas of daily life; improving communication skills and exercising empathy. The development of these skills is planned throughout the entire schooling process from early childhood education to secondary education, distributed among the different areas of knowledge according to the specificities of each of them (MEC, 2018).

Despite the creation of such initiatives, however, there are few developments in this field. Thus, in Argentina particularly, the findings are associated with investigating the relationship between life skills and gender, establishing some differences with adolescents from public schools (Cardozo et al., 2011). Furthermore, the implementation of certain interventions was also observed with public schools, this time with both teachers and students, addressing the problem of drug use, providing useful tools in the construction of educational projects on HpV (Ardiles et al., 2012). Generally, regulations from the National Ministry of Education and provincial governments are implemented with the objective of carrying out tasks to prevent the consumption of psychoactive substances as educational projects based on the life skills strategy (Ministry of Education, 2016). In this way, one of the best-known models at the country level called ESTAR in Prevention (Territorial Space for the Articulation of Networks in Prevention) is presented, which, from the focus of selective prevention, promotes the creation and implementation of the "Being in

Prevention" in the educational units, taking as the axis of its strategy the active participation of the educational community, to collectively address drug consumption. This is a program for formal and non-formal education levels, with the support of the National Education and Prevention Program on Addictions and Drug Abuse of the Ministry of Education and Sports of the Nation, in coordination with other sectors (Secretariat of Comprehensive Policies of the Argentine Nation [SEDRONAR], s/f).

Continuing with the implementation of proposals for interventions in Life Skills in Brazil, the exploratory study carried out by Santos and Carvalho (2021) aimed to describe group interventions aimed at the development of life skills in Brazilian children and adolescents. With a time cut of 20 years (2001–2021), the article included studies in the Portuguese language and carried out in Brazil, based on the definition of HpV according to the WHO and that were intended for children and/or adolescents. The bibliographic research used the Google Scholar database, adjusting the descriptors to "life skills" (life skills), "life skills and children" (life skills and children), "life skills and adolescents" (skills for life and adolescents), using in Portuguese variations of the term that itself also means skills for life: "skills for life and children" and "skills for life and adolescents," selecting eight interventions. The analysis of the results indicated that 75% of the interventions were in public schools, whether from the municipal or state network, being in line with the fact mentioned above about the strategic role of educational institutions in carrying out such activities with students (Vieira et al., 2014). The participants were adolescents between 12 and 18 years old. (75%), with the exception of two studies that included children with a minimum age of 8 years in their samples. The programs are directly or indirectly related to health promotion, paying attention in addition to the development of HpV, to debates on sexuality and gender issues (50%), prevention of risk behaviors and promotion of social skills, present in 37.5% of the interventions. Other topics, such as creating a support network, preventing psychoactive substance use, increasing quality of life, mental health considerations, and the use of Cognitive Behavioral Therapy techniques, were addressed in the 12th, 5% of each of the studies. The results, in general, indicated progress in the aspects worked on, highlighting, for example, the improvement of interpersonal relationships, a greater ability to manage emotions and less exposure to risk behaviors. However, it should be noted that although 75% of the studies have conducted some type of quantitative analysis, data from 33.3% of these interventions indicate inconsistencies in the benefits perceived and reported by participants with respect to the results found after qualitative analysis. It is relevant to note that 62.5% of the interventions occurred in the southeastern region of Brazil, while the remaining 37.5% in the central-western region of the country. Therefore, it is proposed that more quantitative studies should be carried out on HpV interventions aimed at young people and adolescents in Brazil, also taking into account that these projects are evaluated in other regions of the country, especially when considering the diversity of the different Brazilian contexts (Brazilian Ministry of Education, 2018).

By analyzing more specifically the program developed by Murta and collaborators (2013), it can be illustrated how the practice of health promotion in HpV occurs in Brazilian schools. With the aim of acting against dating violence and sexist and homophobic beliefs through the promotion of HpV and sexual and reproductive rights, the authors conducted a study with 60 first-year high school students from a public school in Brasília (DF), aged between 14 and 18 years, who were divided into an intervention group (N = 27) and a control group (N = 33). Initially, the knowledge and beliefs of the students in the first group on topics related to sexuality and sexual and reproductive rights were evaluated, as well as their interests and suggestions regarding the topics to be addressed. Based on the students' considerations, 7 weekly meetings were held, each lasting 80 min, during the school day. The activities had a participatory nature and the sessions were structured in order to evaluate the skills applied during the week, perform and discuss the main technique, propose a homework assignment, and receive comments from the students about the day's meeting. The topics addressed were self-knowledge, critical thinking, assertive communication, empathy, emotion management, decision making, and problem solving. According to the data analyzed by the authors, the adolescents transferred the skills learned in the meetings to their daily lives and, in the case of some participants, these remained active even 5 months after the intervention. Only 25% of the participants stated that they had not noticed any differences in their way of thinking after participating in the program, while 33% reported no differences in their way of acting. The comparison between the intervention and control groups allowed the authors to verify a reduction in overt hostile sexist and homophobic responses in the group that received the intervention, and an increase in non-sexist and non-homophobic responses by these students. However, no significant differences were found in terms of the intention to confront dating violence between the two groups, but both showed improvements in terms of negotiation and ending these situations (Murta et al., 2013).

Despite the recognition of the relevance of HpV development programs for promoting the health of students, it is observed that there are still few Brazilian studies produced. This reality limits a deeper analysis of the possible benefits derived from these programs. On the other hand, there is a growing need to intervene to promote the mental health of children and young people of school age, which gives urgency to the development of actions aimed at guaranteeing the increase of individual and group protection factors (Fernandes et al., 2020; Lopes, 2020; Murta et al., 2015). In this context, initiatives are observed that, although not specifically aimed at promoting HpV, focus on skills considered beneficial for the development of Brazilian youth (Carbogim et al., 2019; Silva et al., 2018), which suggests some agreement between researchers from different areas regarding the positive role of these actions.

Fundamentals of an Intervention in Life Skills for the Prevention of Drug Use in the Educational Field

This Life Skills protocol involved reflecting, as part of the design, on those theoretical principles or key pillars that would define the objectives to be met in its implementation, which tend to contribute in a critical and autonomous decision-making in caring behaviors with oneself and others, thereby reducing the risks associated with drug use. These principles make it possible to monitor the process and final evaluation of compliance with the main factors in the development of Life Skills for young people, establishing a certain coherence between the method and its foundations. The main axis refers to the approach to Life Skills in its three main categories: cognitive, emotional, and social skills. According to the state of the art of scientific literature, the skills used in the field of drug prevention and which were selected for the present intervention correspond primarily to self-knowledge, emotion control and stress management, interpersonal relationships among which empathy and assertiveness, critical thinking and beliefs about drugs are addressed. Although the latter is not integrated as a skill from the WHO concept, various studies include it as a way of delving into the prevention of consumption (Maalouf et al., 2019; Pérez de la Barrera, 2012; Spaeth et al., 2010). Likewise, the life project is established as an essential topic to be discussed in adolescents, prioritizing collective community projects over individual ones in order to be part of and be a protagonist of social transformation, in which the strengthening of ties and Solidarity constitutes pillars for the development of protective factors in community health (Ministry of Education of the Nation & Sedronar, 2021; Pérez de la Barrera, 2012). Conceptually, life skills from the WHO are defined as:

The ability of an individual to effectively meet the demands and challenges of daily life. It is your ability to maintain a state of mental well-being and express it through adaptive and positive behavior in your interactions with others, with your own culture and environment (1993, p. 6).

Such tools promote in young people those conditions to achieve greater psychosocial well-being in coexistence with others in different contexts, strengthening interpersonal ties and solidarity (PAHO & WHO, 2018). Botvin and Kantor (2000) present a model of etiological factors in the consumption of psychoactive substances and how life skills would operate in the prevention of the use of alcohol, tobacco, and other drugs. Therefore, being a multi-determined phenomenon, in which personal, family, and social aspects converge, skills allow the strengthening of competencies to face difficulties, influencing critical knowledge about social regulations regarding drug use; developing the ability to resist peer pressure as personal self-management linked to decision making and emotional control; and social skills to improve interpersonal relationships. In this way, it is presented as a complex model that affects the etiological determinants of drug consumption.

Furthermore, it is necessary to incorporate the Harm Reduction Paradigm as another foundation given that we work with the phenomenon of consumption, it maintains that abstinence is not the ultimate goal and depends on the motivations of each person, recognizing that many of them may not want to abandon their consumption practices (Sedronar, 2019). Faced with this, it is important to carry out health strategies that protect the human rights and well-being of subjects, promoting caring behaviors to minimize risks linked to such practices. The Organization of American States [OAS] (2012) defines harm reduction in the following way: "Notion that brings together policies, programs and practices aimed at mitigating the negative consequences at a social, economic and health level that are due to the consumption of legal and illegal psychoactive drugs, without necessarily reducing said consumption" (p. 16).

To complement these theoretical pillars, concepts are considered that, although they are theoretical developments, they also imply a methodological framework of action for the processes of training and apprehension of skills. The principles of Popular Education were adopted that promote the participation of young people through dialogue, critical reflection, and problematization of reality to consequently develop autonomy in their health processes. Therefore, an axis that runs through the entire intervention is related to the fact that knowledge is not something that is possessed and transferred from the coordinator to the student; on the contrary, it is constructed as a group and transformed (Freire, 1999). It is necessary to take into account that for this construction to occur and not the reproduction of knowledge and/or discourses around care behaviors such as beliefs about drug use, it is essential to enable respect for both the process of critical awareness, which is not generated immediately and, on the other hand, respect for the knowledge that adolescents possess, promoting their ability to problematize and create. A tool that is available to achieve this goal is dialogue, where what is understood is communicated and produced with others.

The coherent task of the educator who thinks correctly is, while exercising as a human being the irrefutable practice of understanding, to challenge the student with whom he communicates and to whom he communicates, to produce his understanding and intercommunication and that is not based on the capacity for dialogue. That is why thinking correctly is dialogic and not polemical (Freire, 1999, p. 39).

Likewise, respect for the autonomy of the subject is incorporated, establishing an ethical relationship with others and equality, not devaluing their beliefs and knowledge in order to promote their curiosity in freedom. To do this, a dialogic relationship is established where the active and inquiring role of the participants is put on stage either by listening or by using the word to ask, question, and approach the understanding of the facts. In this democratization of learning, listening is constituted as an element that favors speaking with the other in this context of dialogue, in order to be able to open up the differences and singularities of the participants without assuming an authoritarian position (Freire, 1999). These instruments contribute to understanding the diversity of positions regarding drug use and, within the group, to be able to develop knowledge that does not minimize the perceptions of others, but rather enriches their view of the phenomenon or even generates questions without offering complete and clear answers.

Based on the conceptual journey carried out, this chapter proposes to understand the bases that support the way of thinking about education in life skills with adolescents and to reflect on the possibilities of applying such principles in a pilot protocol for the prevention of use of psychoactive substances in the educational context. The challenges and/or limitations of this approach are discussed, as well as the facilitating and potentializing aspects in the health promotion process necessary to be strengthened in future applications of the intervention.

Characteristics of the Pilot Application with Adolescents and Young People in Argentina and Brazil

In accordance with the adaptation process of the initially constructed protocol, it was carried out in educational institutions in both Argentina and Brazil, taking into account its particularities according to the context and characteristics of the adolescents. It is presented how access to the field was and the singularities of each of the groups which enriched the teams way of thinking about life skills training, making the proposals first developed more flexible.

The design of the group objectives and techniques that make up the Life Skills protocol were developed based on information from the portals of the Ministry of Health of the Argentine Nation, SEDRONAR and international organizations that deal with the aforementioned work. Techniques were chosen that work on each skill in a playful and reflective way, enabling group interaction rather than individual interaction.

During the year 2021, in the month of November, the pilot test of the protocol was carried out in a town located in a province in northern Argentina, in a context where we were moving towards the post-COVID-19 pandemic and presence in schools was possible. The field of intervention selected was for convenience since it is the place of origin of one of the team members, facilitating entry to the educational institution to carry out the work, the said school was characterized by being of technical education. The director was open to the proposal, providing the space for activities with students between 15 and 17 years old. At that time, we worked with the morning and afternoon shift, with two homogeneous groups since they belonged to the same classroom, varying the participation between 11 and 14 adolescents. The selection of the participants was in accordance with the director's instructions, which could be incorporated into the tasks with motivation and also due to the need for an intervention with one of the groups. However, during the meetings the voluntariness of their participation was clearly expressed. In this period, they were studying the last week of the school year, so some meetings were held with the morning shift, where the majority of the students had to complete the practice activities during the afternoon, thus having greater time availability; and the others with the late shift to be able to finish the pilot intervention given that the main objective was to evaluate the techniques and methodology used. Therefore, the topic on self-knowledge and control of emotions and stress was carried out with the students of the double shift, continuing on the same day with the two workshops; and finally the life project. Themes linked to interpersonal relationships, empathy, and assertiveness such as critical thinking and beliefs about drugs were developed with the afternoon group on two consecutive days. Such groups were characterized by belonging to different socioeconomic and cultural sectors, which influenced the autonomy of group participation. From the results, the need to readapt the protocol according to school time was evident, varying from 40 to 60 min; initially it was designed for a period of 2 h. Most of the meetings were carried out during free hours, presenting as an obstacle the time available to finish the meetings, and a weekly meeting was previously planned, it took place after 3 days, which in terms of impact of the intervention in young people would be an aspect to analyze later. Likewise, in terms of the proposed dynamic, it was necessary to give more space to the words, desires, and needs of young people, building an environment different from traditional classes, being less expository and more participatory at times.

Another challenge was with one of the groups, starting with simple activities advancing in complexity, requiring the support of the coordinator given that according to the group process, work in small groups and individually was not possible. Regarding the space offered, the two groups expressed its importance and the need for its continuity in the institution due to conflicts with the adult figure (managers and teachers) as well as the desire to strengthen themselves as a group after the pandemic period. They valued the opportunity to express themselves and be heard discussing topics that are not usually discussed in classes with teachers. A bond was established between the students and the coordinator throughout the process that, although it was brief, demonstrating in each meeting motivation and interest in the tasks and in their completion, they requested to take one of the cards used as a souvenir, a technique for addressing beliefs about drugs, as well as one of the students gave the coordinator a paper with his signature to remember it. Likewise, prior to each workshop, the students were already arranged in a circle as part of the group device initially adopted. In this first approach to the group under study, as the objective was to evaluate the protocol, neither the Life Skills scales nor those to identify problematic substance use were administered.

In the Brazilian context, the implementation experience of the pilot project took place with students recently admitted to the Psychology course at the Federal University of Juiz de Fora, known as "calouros." The activity was titled "Strengthening bonds and skills for life: support for Psychology 2022 entrants." So that the project could be implemented, a first contact was made with the course coordination, even before the start of the school year, as a way to present it and verify the viability of offering it to new students. After the coordination was accepted, the call was prepared, containing the main information on the axes to be discussed, as well as the dates, places, and times of the activities. The invitation was disseminated through the research group's social networks and shared through the students' WhatsApp. Registrations were through an electronic Google form that collected basic information about interested students, investigating their expectations about the meetings. All participants signed the informed consent form.

Although 11 students were initially registered, only 8 attended the first meeting, a number that remained stable over time. The sample was made up of 6 females and 2 males, 75% of the subjects were between 17 and 18 years old. The other 2 participants, aged 23 and 30, were considered given that the objective of the intervention of providing support for the entrants was respected. The motivations for joining the group were diverse, observing that the common factor lies in the importance of feeling contained during this new phase of life, which was characterized by going through a period of social isolation due to the COVID-19 pandemic. Entering university meant the need to generate new adaptive strategies because a large part of the young people migrated to Juiz de Fora to begin their higher studies.

The proposal was that each meeting would last 1 h. However, the students requested an extension of an hour and a half, to be able to delve deeper into the topics. The activities began with an ice-breaking technique and/or a relaxation technique, in which the participants tended to get very involved, showing that they were having fun, signifying a break from everyday life. Subsequently, the group was introduced for the maintenance exercise, in which the reflections and actions carried out by the students during the week were discussed, based on the debates held in the previous meeting. In general, these were moments in which the young people reported on the way in which they were applying the topics in their daily lives, highlighting personal moments in which the issues discussed in the group were useful for better handling the situations they faced with each other. The tendency to share personal issues required the coordinators to be able to establish a parallel between the narrated events and the group discussion, in order to guarantee that the process had as its axis group enrichment to the detriment of individual analysis of the situations. In this way, the group was able to benefit from the individual experiences of the participants as a way to consolidate collective learning.

The group showed commitment during the execution of the main techniques. The proposed topics were explored through group discussions arranged in a circle, in which participants were invited to share their impressions, listen to the position of their colleagues and think about ways to resolve the proposed situations based on the use of skills to life, especially those discussed on the day of the meeting. A certain group autonomy was observed in the conduct of the dialogues, which occurred in an articulated manner, establishing parallels between the topics worked on and the experiences of the subjects in question. It was up to the facilitators to collaborate with the orientation of the discussions, in order to guarantee that all students had a moment to speak according to their interests, in addition to seeking a theoretical and experiential depth in relation to the topic of each meeting. In this sense, group dynamics techniques adapted to the context in question were adopted as a way to offer a starting point for debates and encourage student participation. At the end of the meetings, students were asked to make a list of words that summarized the day's activities, as a way to bring an emotional closure to the meeting. The observations derived from each of the days were recorded in the field diaries of the coordinators, who subsequently shared their notes with each other, forming a framework of impressions and experiences with respect to the pilot group.

The conduct of the activities was affected by specific situations in the educational field. In this context, the need to extend the period of interventions was highlighted, caused both by the unavailability of students during their exam period and by the increase in the number of COVID-19 cases among psychology teachers and students, which was reflected in an addition of 3 weeks to the initial schedule. It was decided that one of the meetings would be held through the Google Meet platform. This situation had a direct impact on the level of participation of the students, since, despite the attempt to transfer and adapt the proposed dynamics to the virtual environment, a large part of the young people did not turn on the cameras, using the chat to speak, reducing spontaneity of the interventions. At the end of this meeting, the coordinators and students maintained the importance of giving priority to in-person meetings, even if this implied a new organization of the calendar.

As a way to evaluate the results of the intervention, in the first meeting the following were applied: the Life Skills Scale and the Alcohol, Tobacco, and Other Substance Use Detection Test (ASSIST), as well as three questions from the Alcohol Use Disorders Identification (AUDIT). The participants showed interest in answering the proposed questionnaires, staying focused on the activity and, on some occasions, exchanging impressions among themselves about their own answers. It was highlighted that the instruments provided a moment of self-knowledge and reflection on the consumption of psychoactive substances, which can impact the way in which subjects perceive their individual position in relation to everyday issues and, more specifically, their behaviors in relation to the consumption of alcohol and other drugs. Four weeks after the last meeting, the Life Skills Scale was repeated, which took place at different times with the participants due to the difficulty of reconciling everyone's schedule.

Throughout the process, student assessment was crucial for the team to better understand what modifications would be relevant to make the intervention more efficient and appropriate. In this sense, the participants were asked for their opinion on the development of the activities, highlighting the relevance of this action for better planning and execution of the program in its subsequent applications. As students provided contributions, the team worked to incorporate them, such as asking for more time to complete activities and prioritizing in-person meetings. In the last meeting, a more systematized evaluation process was developed, in which the group was asked to indicate their impressions about the topics worked on, the techniques used, the time spent on each activity, and the conduct of the facilitators. In general, the assessments made indicated reinforcing the group space as a favorable environment for welcome and reflection, as well as for the creation of links both between colleagues and between them and the coordinators. The creation of a space in which they felt heard and respected in their opinions was highlighted, guaranteeing a comfortable and safe environment. Finally, the dynamic implemented was praised and a longer execution time was suggested, to ensure that they had greater exploration of their potential and a more robust closure of their discussion.

Evaluation of the Proposed Methodology and Preliminary Results of the Process with Young People: Challenges and Potentialities

Taking into account that these were pilot interventions, through which it was intended to evaluate both the viability of the project and its possible benefits, the analysis of the results presented here focused on critically reflecting on the impacts of the implemented activities. In this sense, we start from the considerations that were reported by the participants throughout the process, articulating them with the team's impressions—which were recorded in field diaries—, producing a qualitative analysis of the results described above, as a way of analyzing objectively the experience and learning involved in the implementation of the project so far, in order to improve the following practices.

Regarding the methodology, one of the criteria refers to the way in which the students were called to participate in the project, understanding that there were positive aspects and others to be rethought. As for the Argentine pilot group, a prior call was not made, but based on the director's considerations, the groups were selected, given that as they were close to the end of the school year, some of the other courses were not attending the school. A presentation was made on the topics to be addressed and the young people expressed interest in being part of the project. Faced with this scenario, when analyzing the impact of the actions carried out, it is highlighted that only some meetings were held with a group in the morning and others in the afternoon, not offering the sequence of the five meetings to each one, which is considered a difficulty in the process. For this reason, it is emphasized to take into account the school's schedule and to know in advance the group's object of intervention, showing their motivations to participate, forming the groups based on their own interests beyond the perspective of the directors of the institution, although they expressed the voluntariness of participation.

In the Brazilian experience, the use of social networks to publicize the program turned out to be an interesting tool, since it required less time on the part of the organizers when compared to an invitation made in person, which would require greater procedures in terms of the availability of time and travel to contact students. On the other hand, to fulfill the purpose of promoting the creation of links between first-year students, the dissemination of the project took place right at the beginning of classes, which may have influenced the number of students who actually had access to the invitation and, therefore, in the possibility of all interested parties participating. An attempt was made to remedy this situation by asking the course coordination and students from later periods to collaborate in disseminating the activity. In any case, it is important to have more time to actively generate dissemination to students on future occasions, since greater care in this initial phase can influence the participants' adherence to the proposed action (Lopes et al., 2014).

Certainly, although it was an extracurricular activity, in which participation was voluntary, in both groups the number of participants remained stable from start to finish, which suggests a true disposition towards the topics worked on. It is observed that although, in the case of secondary students, the project was developed during school hours and their presence could have been influenced by class attendance, the decision to be present at the meetings, participating according to their possibilities, was already clear that some students had to withdraw to take retakes of the subjects. In each of the meetings, the students were invited to express their impressions about the actions developed, in order to understand which aspects contribute to the group's adhesion and which should be reformulated to make the process more attractive to the public. In this context, the horizontality of the relationships was pointed out as a positive point, since the participants expressed feeling contemplated when attending a space in which their word was not only respected but also requested, expressing feelings of tranquility and relief when being able to express what they thought and felt. The dynamism of the process was also pointed out as an attractive factor by the young people, who praised, at different times, the proposed tasks in terms of their potential to provoke general participation in a relaxed way. The adoption of topics considered relevant by the recipients, associated with a participatory approach to the activities, is in line with what is established by Popular Education, which emphasizes the need to value the active role of the subjects in their training process, based on concrete demands that generate enriching discussions about ways of life (Freire, 1999).

Taking into account the dynamics developed, it is worth highlighting that more time was requested to carry them out, in order to allow greater reflection on the complex issues that were addressed, as well as to enable the strengthening of the bond between adolescents given the pandemic period they were going through. In fact, the question of time is something that must be considered with caution, some studies report that to achieve effects on the development of skills, the duration of the interventions should be longer, and longitudinal measurements should be carried out (Morales et al., 2013). In turn, Maalouf et al. (2019) provide that the number of sessions is not a crucial factor in itself to achieve the desired effects, but rather it is necessary to have well-defined objectives and implement them efficiently to achieve the expected changes in skills. Despite this, the educational context has particularities that require certain flexibility on the part of the team so that the process is fruitful for those involved. In the Brazilian context, it was possible to adapt the meeting schedule based on student demand, which was not equally executed in the Argentine school context due to the same limitations of the school schedule and institutional dynamics, taking into account that the project was developed in the students' free hours. According to the team's experience, it is possible to reach the conclusion that in school reality, working with adolescents requires a series of agreements, which imply, for example, the granting of physical space by school staff; the availability of schedules to hold the meetings, which, in some cases, must be negotiated directly with the teachers; and the authorization of those responsible for the participation of activities during extracurricular hours in the case of minors. Furthermore, adversities related to everyday situations—such as student exam week or the worsening of COVID cases, for example— have a direct impact on the organization of the project, which is reflected in the availability of hours reserved for carrying out each of the activities. Thus, based on the team's observations of the situations faced in the interventions described here, it is understood that some measures can be adopted to minimize unforeseen events in the schedule, as well as to make better use of the intervention periods, such as previously investigating the availability of schedules of the subjects interested in the project; establish agreements with the school team on the dates and duration of activities; create a means of communication with participants as a way to transmit notices about schedule changes and receive information about the need for absences; and propose a schedule that is realistic and adaptable, considering the need to replan actions in the event of possible circumstantial situations.

Considerations on the most general aspects of the protocol related to the language, content, and modality of the intervention (Manzini, 2004) were evaluated satisfactorily by the groups, in addition to its novelty in terms of the dynamics adopted that differ from the traditional class format, giving value to the participation of the adolescent. A space was offered for suggestions where they expressed that in addition to the techniques used, they would like to incorporate talks on specific topics related to anxiety, sadness, and mental health since they are not aspects that are generally raised during classes with teachers. On the other hand, they expressed activities of interest to be included in the meetings such as playing games, listening to music of their choice, making drawings, art, sharing a drink or food that impact the development of bonds and getting to know each other with their peers. Regarding the planning of proposed activities, they commented on continuing with relaxation and/or meditation exercises, and the use of posters or blackboards since it facilitates understanding of the topics. Particularly, the role of the coordinator played by the team members was valued positively since the slogans and conceptual references were presented in an entertaining, explanatory, and appropriate manner according to the audience to which they were directed. Group participation was another item to be evaluated, the adolescents valued the importance of the topic and that it would have been more beneficial if more students had joined the project, referring to the fact that their other classmates did not attend the meetings to generate more rich debates. Their participation was valued as positive given that they managed to reflect, listen to their partner, express their opinions, as well as adapt to group work.

On the other hand, those results associated with the effects of the intervention in young people from both samples are evident when apprehending life skills as well as their perspectives on their practice. The findings are grouped according to each of the encounters, graphing with their words the relevance of what was learned, as well as some problems that arose.

In the first meeting on self-knowledge, the difficulty in identifying their own tastes, preferences, and unique characteristics that differentiated them was observed. The activity carried out to reflect on this thematic axis involved a collage on such characteristics, as a result, it was evident that the productions were kept to oneself without sharing with others, causing shame and not exposing oneself to the gaze of others. These analyses were verbalized by themselves, affirming the need and importance of developing one's own knowledge. Participant 1 referred to the "difficulty in seeing ourselves as we are," while subject 2 expressed that "we need to practice these topics, we don't have much self-knowledge."

Thoughts arose during the development of the technique: "Who am I?" as stated by participant 3; just as these graphic productions contributed to thinking more about their strengths than weaknesses, according to participant 4, "it helped me get to know myself in a different way."

In the second workshop on emotion and stress control, both groups experienced some difficulty in recognizing their own emotions, not being able to label or name the emotion experienced physically. At the same time, when dealing with the modalities of coping with emotions, generally the strategies adopted did not correspond to resolving the conflict in an adaptive way, prioritizing avoidance by resorting to carrying out other activities to avoid thinking. Among the coping modalities, crying, aggressiveness or, on the contrary, not reacting, avoiding conflict, stand out, while others placed meditating as that time to mediate the action, or smoking to calm down, and accessing the use of social networks or other cell phone applications to escape from the problem.

Likewise, in the third meeting on interpersonal relationships, specifically the use of empathy and assertiveness; the young people discussed strategies to deal with loneliness, love, and how assertiveness would enable a more supportive and respectful bond with others, valuing knowing what is different since it is more complex when empathizing with one's partner. Furthermore, empathy was defined by subject 5 and participant 6 as "the rights of the other" and "assertiveness as my rights".

In the fourth meeting about critical thinking and beliefs about drugs, young people from both countries agreed that the use of alcohol and other drugs does not resolve conflicts, on the contrary, they aggravate them; these being both emotional and physical health risks. In this direction, they delved into the motivations of the subjects to consume and concluded that there is generally a problem behind it, a cause of a different nature depending on the life history of the subject, using the drug as an escape from their ills or resistance. They also considered strategies to face these difficulties, with psychological or psychiatric therapy being the most relevant. Thus, subject 7 maintained that "many times the person suffers a lot of pressure, so they look for some type of escape valve, whether isolating themselves or taking drugs."

Finally, in the fifth life project meeting, when working on the adult perspective regarding youth, a conflict was observed in the relationship with elders since, in secondary adolescents, they feel obliged to fulfill their study tasks, as well as the hygiene of one's own body. The negative view of adults as "lost, failed, idiotic" young people according to adolescents 8, 9, and 10, implying a lack of respect and understanding for adolescents when they say so. For their part, the young university students maintained that adults trivialize their children's choices and/or decisions, for example, around sexuality, as if it were a passing phase, not valuing the power of decision. Participant 11 graphs what was said in the following way, "parents have difficulty giving autonomy, respecting others, seeing them as subjects." Faced with these conceptions, the participants, when questioned about these perceptions, expressed that they can identify themselves as people who are supportive, who can change the world, offering their children an education different from the one they received; realizing the relevance of educating from childhood in life skills and during all stages of the life cycle to develop healthy relationships with others, as expressed by participant 12, "it is possible to educate throughout life to be top."

Based on the analyses carried out through what was expressed by the adolescents, it is concluded that it is essential to understand them as active subjects not only in the search for academic knowledge but also when prioritizing their concerns and desires, working in proximity with adults through behaviors and support in conflict resolution for the prevention of risk behaviors.

Discussion and Conclusion

The study developed so far allowed us to analyze the pilot test carried out in different contexts—Argentina and Brazil—and involving samples with different characteristics—high school and university students—addressing the possible benefits such as the common and specific factors that need to be altered for the project to be more effective in your next applications. We reflect on the relevance of paying attention to the specificities of the target audience, but without neglecting the factors intrinsic to a well-developed intervention, which imply adequate planning focused on the understandability, attractiveness, and feasibility of the implementation, as well as an adaptability to possible reformulations in the initial project and a deliberative nature regarding the crucial factors for implementation. Thus, we insist on the need to evaluate the social validity of the proposed intervention, in order to investigate whether the actions were relevant from the point of view of their objectives and procedures, guaranteeing the acceptability of the subjects involved and contributing to social transformation of the intended space (Murta & Santos, 2015).

In accordance with what was presented in the investigations of Murta et al. (2013), and Santos and Carvalho (2021), the participants in the interventions reported here indicated that they had noticed improvements in their communication skills, relationships with others, empathy and self-knowledge, aspects that were addressed throughout the meetings. The students identified situations in which it was possible to transfer the knowledge built in the group to their daily lives, highlighting the relevance of carrying out projects in which life skills are presented in a dialogic and reflective way, so that they are incorporated in a meaningful way in the lives of young people.

The limitations of the study include the need for a quantitative analysis of the changes produced in life skills and to be able to compare them with both samples. However, since the scales were not administered in one of the groups, it was not possible to identify such characteristics as the level of consumption observed in the adolescent population. The research was mainly aimed at adapting the protocol and teaching methodology, obtaining qualitative results and an approximation of the possible effects of the intervention.

It is concluded that the interventions in question could contribute, on the one hand, to a better understanding of the potential of the life skills project for the prevention of drug use in the school context and, on the other hand, to the aspects that should be improved for better implementation of the program in schools. Among the factors learned is the importance of investing greater efforts in inviting students to participate in the project, establishing an effective communication channel with the young participants and proposing a realistic calendar of activities adjusted to the availability of the students and the school. Facilitating resources include accessibility to the terrain, configuring a horizontal relationship between the team and participants, and encouraging the sharing of opinions on the functioning of the activities. In this way, we hope to jointly build a program aware of the local reality and committed to socially relevant and contextually viable actions.

Finally, in order to rethink institutional spaces, it is argued that promoting health education requires much more than an isolated intervention with young people; it is crucial to implement the regulations related to carrying out promotional actions for a healthy coexistence and socio-emotional well-being as part of the institutional project, covering not only as a discipline to be taught but also developing actions sustained over time (PAHO & WHO, 2018). In this sense, it refers to the fact that the institution has the capacity to influence the quality of life of its members and it is essential that the interventions to be carried out integrate all dimensions of the environment, training teaching and non-teaching staff, students, parents and incorporating intersectorality to work together with the school and other community and health institutions, expressing the commitment to promote comprehensive health practices for young people (PAHO & WHO, 2018; Sedronar s/f).

References

Ardiles, R., Cardozo, G., Dubini, P., & Fantino, I. E. (2012). Potenciando el autocuidado de la salud en los adolescentes. *Rev. Electrónica sobre extensión universitaria* (3), 1-9. Recuperado de https://perio.unlp.edu.ar/ojs/index.php/extensionenred/article/view/1157

Botvin, G. J., & Kantor, L. W. (2000). Preventing Alcohol and Tobacco use through Life Skills Training. *Alcohol Research & Health, (24)*4, pp. 250-257. Disponible en https://www.ncbi.nlm.nih.gov/pmc/articles/PMC6709746/pdf/arcr-24-4-250.pdf

Carbogim, F.C., Oliveira, L.B., Toledo, M.M., Diaz, F.B.B.S., Bittencourt, G.K.G.D., & Püschel, V.A.A. (2019). Active teaching model to promote critical thinking. *Rev Bras Enferm 72*(1), 293-8. https://doi.org/10.1590/0034-7167-2018-0002

Cardozo, G., Dubini, P., Fantino, I., & Ardiles, R. (2011). Habilidades para la vida en adolescentes: Diferencias de género, correlaciones entre habilidades y variables predictoras de la empatía. *Psicología desde el Caribe*, *28*, 107-132. SciELO Colombia. https://www.redalyc.org/articulo.oa?id=21320758006

Comisión económica para américa latina y el caribe (2022, 5 de setiembre). *Juventud.* CEPAL, 2022. Disponível em: https://www.cepal.org/es/subtemas/juventud#

Fernandes, F. Y., Freitas, B. H. B. M., Marcon, S. R., Arruda, V. L., Lima, N. V. P., Bortolini, J., & Gaíva, M. A. M. (2020). Tendência de suicídio em adolescentes brasileiros entre 1997 e 2016. *Epidemiologia e Serviços de Saúde 29*(4), 1-10. https://doi.org/10.1590/S1679-49742020000400025.

Fondo de las Naciones Unidas para la Infancia (2021). *Salud mental en tiempos de coronavirus.* Disponible en: https://www.unicef.org/argentina/media/12106/file/Estudio%20sobre%20los%20efectos%20en%20la%20salud%20mental%20de%20ni%C3%B1as,%20ni%C3%B1os%20y%20adolescentes%20por%20COVID-19.pdf

Fondo de las Naciones Unidas para la Infancia (2022, 5 de diciembre). *Saúde mental de adolescentes. A pandemia reforçou a urgência de medidas para garantir o bem-estar de toda uma geração.* [Comunicado de prensa]. Disponible en https://www.unicef.org/brazil/saude-mental-de-adolescentes

Fondo de las Naciones Unidas para la Infancia (2022, 5 de diciembre). *Metade dos adolescentes e jovens sentiu necessidade de pedir ajuda em relação à saúde mental recentemente, mostra enquete do UNICEF com a Viração.* [Comunicado de prensa]. Disponible en https://www.unicef.org/brazil/comunicados-de-imprensa/metade-dos-adolescentes-e-jovens-sentiu-necessidade-de-pedir-ajuda-em-relacao-a-saude-mental-recentemente

Freire, P. (1999). *Pedagogía de la autonomía. Saberes necesarios para la práctica educativa*. Ed. Siglo XXI.

Instituto Brasileño de Geografía y Estadística (2021, 10 de setiembre). *Seis em cada dez estudantes haviam experimentado bebida alcoólica na pré-pandemia.* [Comunicado de prensa]. Disponible en https://agenciadenoticias.ibge.gov.br/agencia-noticias/2012-agencia-de-noticias/noticias/31580-seis-em-cada-dez-estudantes-haviam-experimentado-bebida-alcoolica-na-pre-pandemia

Lopes, C. S. (2020). Como está a saúde mental dos brasileiros? A importância das coortes de nascimento para melhor compreensão do problema. *Cadernos de Saúde Pública 36*(2), 1-4. https://doi.org/10.1590/0102-311X00005020.

Lopes, F. M., Peuker, A. C. W. B., Rech, B. E., Gonçalves, R. & Bizarro, L. (2014). Desenvolvimento, divulgação, adesão e eficácia de um Programa de Cessação do Tabagismo oferecido em uma universidade pública. *Cadernos Brasileiros De Terapia Ocupacional, 22*(1SE). https://doi.org/10.4322/cto.2014.025

Maalouf, W., Stojanovic, M., Kiefer, M., Campello, G., Heikkila, H., & El-Khatib, Z. (2019). Lions Quest Skills for Adolescence Program as a School Intervention to Prevent Substance Use-a Pilot Study Across Three South East European Countries. *Prevention Science: The Official Journal of the Society for Prevention Research, 20*(4), 555-565. https://doi.org/10.1007/s11121-019-01012-6

Manzini, E. (2004): Entrevista semi-estruturada: Análise de objetivos e de roteiros. Em Seminário Internacional sobre pesquisa e estudos qualitativos, 2, 2004, Bauru. A pesquisa qualitativa em debate. Anais Bauru: USC, 2004. CD-ROOM. ISBN:85-98623-01-6. 10p.

Ministerio de Educación. Brasil. (2018). Base Nacional Comum Curricular. Brasília. Disponible en http://basenacionalcomum.mec.gov.br/

Ministerio de Educación. Brasil (1997). Parâmetros curriculares nacionais: introdução aos parâmetros curriculares nacionais. Disponible en http://portal.mec.gov.br/seb/arquivos/pdf/livro01.pdf

Ministerio de Educación, Neuquén, Argentina (2018). *Convivencias escolares. Notas para pensar los modos de habitar las escuelas.* Recuperado de: https://www.neuquen.edu.ar/wp-content/uploads/2016/08/CUADERNILLO-1.pdf

Ministerio de Educación, Neuquén, Argentina (2016). *Prevención de las adicciones y consumos problemáticos de sustancias.* Recuperado de https://www.neuquen.edu.ar/wp-content/uploads/2016/08/PUBLICACION_ADICCIONES.pdf4

Ministerio de Educación de la Nación & Secretaría de Políticas Integrales de la Nación Argentina (2021). *Tomá la voz: ejes y propuestas para el abordaje de los consumos problemáticos en el ámbito educativo.* Ciud. Autónoma de Buenos Aires.

Ministerio de Salud, Argentina (11 de agosto de 2021). Salud impulsa la Estrategia Nacional de Entornos Saludables. Disponible en: https://www.argentina.gob.ar/noticias/salud-impulsa-la-estrategia-nacional-de-entornos-saludables

Ministerio de Salud Argentina (2021). *ENES-ES. Escuelas saludables.* Recuperado de: http://servicios.infoleg.gob.ar/infolegInternet/anexos/350000-354999/352776/res2198-2.pdf

Morales, M., Benítez, M., & Agustín, D. (2013). Habilidades para la vida (cognitivas y sociales) en adolescentes de una zona rural. *Revista Electrónica de Investigación Educativa, 15*(3), 98-113. Recuperado de http://redie.uabc.mx/vol15no3/contenido-moralesetal.html

Murta, S. G., Günther, I. A., & Guzzo, R. S. L. (2015). Prevenção e promoção em saúde mental no curso de vida: indicadores para a ação. In: S. G. Murta, C. Leandro-França, K. B. Santos & L. Polejack (Orgs.). *Prevenção e promoção em saúde mental* (pp. 75-92). Novo Hamburgo: Sinopsys.

Murta, S. G., & Santos, K. B. (2015). Desenvolvimento de programas preventivos e de promoção de saúde mental. In: S. G. Murta, C. Leandro-França, K. B. Santos & L. Polejack (Orgs.). *Prevenção e promoção em saúde mental* (pp. 168-191). Novo Hamburgo: Sinopsys.

Murta, S. G., Santos, B. R. P., Nobre, L. A., Araújo, I. F., Miranda, A. A. V., Rodrigues, I. O., & Franco, C. T. P. (2013). Prevenção à violência no namoro e promoção de habi-

lidades de vida em adolescentes. *Psicologia USP 24*(2), 263-288. https://doi.org/10.1590/S0103-65642013000200005.
Organización de los Estados Americanos (2012). *Escenarios para el problema de drogas en las Américas 2013-2025.* Recuperado de: https://idpc.net/es/publications/2013/05/informe-de-la-oea-escenarios-para-el-problema-de-drogas-en-las-americas-2013-2025
Organización Mundial de la Salud. (1993). *Enseñanza en los colegios de las habilidades para vivir.* Recuperado de: http://centroderecursos.alboan.org/ebooks/0000/0148/Ense%C3%B1anza_en_los_colegios_de_las_habilidades_para_la_vida.pdf
Organización Mundial de la Salud (30 de octubre de 2022). *Salud mental del adolescente.* OMS 2021. Recuperado de https://www.who.int/es/news-room/fact-sheets/detail/adolescent-mental-health
Organización Panamericana de la Salud (30 de octubre de 2022). *Estado de salud de la población. La salud mental en la Región de las Américas 2017.* OPS. Recuperado de https://www.paho.org/salud-en-las-americas-2017/ro-mental-es.html
Organización Panamericana de Salud & Organización Mundial de la Salud (2018). *Promover la salud en la escuela. ¿Cómo construir una escuela promotora de salud?.* Recuperado de: https://iris.paho.org/bitstream/handle/10665.2/49146/OPSARG18031-spa.pdf?sequence=1&isAllowed=y
Pan-American Life (2022). Salud mental en América Latina y el Caribe. La pandemia silenciosa. Recuperado de https://www.palig.com/Media/Default/Documents/Salud%20Mental%20White%20Paper%20PALIG.pdf
Pérez de la Barrera, C. (2012). Habilidades para la vida y consumo de drogas en adolescentes escolarizados mexicanos. *Adicciones, 24*(2), 153-160. https://doi.org/10.20882/adicciones.108
Santos, K. B., & Carvalho, A.L.N. (2021). Intervenções em habilidades de vida: contribuições para o desenvolvimento psicossocial de crianças e adolescentes. *Rev. Bras. Psico. e Educ., 22*, pp. 1-12. https://periodicos.fclar.unesp.br/doxa/article/download/15349/11780/52248
Secretaría de Políticas Integrales de la Nación Argentina (s/f): *Estar en prevención. Espacio territorial de articulación de redes en prevención.* Recuperado de http://www.prevencionenadicciones.unsl.edu.ar/Estar%20en%20Prevencion.pdf
Secretaría de Políticas Integrales de la Nación Argentina (s/f.). *Orientación para la intervención. Guía de orientación para la intervención en situaciones de consumo problemático de sustancias en la escuela.*
Secretaría de Políticas Integrales de la Nación Argentina (2019). *Manual de estrategias preventivas en contextos de ocio nocturno y recreativos. Pasala mejor. Más cuidados menos riesgos.* Recuperado de: https://www.argentina.gob.ar/sites/default/files/manual_nocturnidad_final.pdf
Silva, J. L., Oliveira, W. A., Carlos, D. M., Lizzi, E. A. S., Rosário, R., Silva, M. A. I. (2018). Intervention in Social Skills and Bullying. *Revista Brasileira de Enfermagem 71*(3), 1085-1091. https://doi.org/10.1590/0034-7167-2017-0151
Spaeth, M., Weichold, K., Silbereisen, R. K., & Wiesner, M. (2010). Examining the differential effectiveness of a life skills program (IPSY) on alcohol use trajectories in early adolescence. *Journal of Consulting and Clinical Psychology, 78*(3), 334-348. https://doi.org/10.1037/a0019550
Vieira, M. A., Estanislau, G. M., Bressan, R. A., & Bodin, I. A. (2014). Saúde mental na escola. In Estanislau, G. M. & Bressan, R. A. (Orgs.). *Saúde mental na escola: o que os educadores devem saber* (pp. 13-23). Porto Alegre: Artmed.

María Elena Iturriaga Goroso is a Psychologist from Universidad Nacional de Tucumán (UNT), Argentina. Master's degree and PhD in Psychology from the Universidade Federal de Juiz de Fora (UFJF), Brazil. Researcher of the Center for Research, Intervention and Evaluation in Alcohol and Drugs (CREPEIA) of UFJF and Áncora Research Group (UNT).

Thaís Soares Pereira is a Psychologist from the Universidade Federal de Juiz de Fora (UFJF), Brazil. Master's student in Psychology at UFJF. Member of the Center for Research, Intervention and Evaluation for Alcohol & Drugs (CREPEIA-UFJF). Editorial team member of the journal Psicologia em Pesquisa (UFJF).

Telmo Mota Ronzani is a Psychologist, Master's degree in Social Psychology from the Federal University of Minas Gerais (UFMG), PhD from the Federal University of São Paulo (UNIFESP). Postdoctoral researcher at the University of São Paulo (USP) and at the University of Connecticut Health Center (UCHC) in the field of alcohol and other drugs. Full Professor and Vice-President at the Universidade Federal de Juiz de Fora (UFJF), Brazil. Editor-in-Chief of the International Journal of Mental Health and Addiction. Researcher of the Center for Research, Intervention and Evaluation in Alcohol and Drugs (CREPEIA) of UFJF. Scholarship PQ-1 CNPq.

A Systematic View of the Evaluation of Prevention Programs in the Twenty-First Century

Orlando Scoppetta

Introduction

Prevention programs are often the basis of interventions to reduce the incidence of disorders and diseases. The programs, for their part, are built from theories about how disturbances to health and well-being are produced and maintained, from which a set of interventions are provided that are expected to reduce the probability of such disturbances appearing.

However, the internal rationality of a prevention program is a necessary but not sufficient condition for its effectiveness. Therefore, the evaluation of prevention programs constitutes a fundamental pillar in the application of knowledge to achieve greater health and well-being. It is not possible to know if a program is truly preventive if there is no reliable and valid information about its results. Information with these characteristics is called evidence and obtaining evidence about a program is a process that requires time and effort. Additionally, evaluation is a field of practical knowledge that has evolved from strictly summative approaches to more comprehensive ones about program results and the explanation of these results.

The following chapter presents a discussion of the importance of program evaluation as an essential component of prevention. In a way, it is supported that a program without evaluation may be a program, but not a prevention one. In the exposition it is argued that the evaluation of programs is a process inherent to the program itself and that at the same time gives it its intervention credentials that serve the purposes of prevention. The types of evaluation are described according to the purpose and it is shown how a program can have different levels of evidence.

O. Scoppetta (✉)
Research and Evaluation, Corporación Nuevos Rumbos, Bogotá, Colombia
e-mail: oscoppetta@nuevosrumbos.org

A. Pérez-Gómez, J. Mejía-Trujillo (eds.), *Drug Abuse Prevention*, Advances in Mental Health and Addiction, https://doi.org/10.1007/978-3-031-99621-4_9

Likewise, evaluation trends in the twenty-first century are shown and a complementary approach to current approaches is presented.

Evaluation and Rights to Health and Wellbeing

Evaluation is a key component to ensuring that preventive programs work. The purpose of prevention is to reduce the probability of an outcome that affects health and well-being. In the case of drug use, prevention is aimed at avoiding the consumption of harmful substances, especially when it comes to minors, or at reducing the negative results of this practice.

When a person becomes ill or suffers from a preventable behavioral disorder, their treatment and recovery are costly in money, suffering, and loss of quality of life. Many diseases and disorders are preventable and are related to behavior, but changing behavior is not a simple matter. For example, it was in 1954, 70 years ago, when Dr. Richard Doll published "The Mortality of Doctors in Relation to Their Smoking Habits" (Doll & Hill, 1954). Since then, there is increasingly solid evidence that tobacco smoking is associated with multiple diseases and, yet, many people in the world smoke.

Given the complexity of behavioral change to achieve better health, over time an interdisciplinary field developed with important contributions from behavioral sciences, public health, and epidemiology, to name a few. This interdisciplinary field, in turn, gave rise to what is today called the science of prevention. Prevention science is a multidisciplinary scientific field that covers the study of aspects related to the etiology, epidemiology, design, effectiveness, and implementation of preventive interventions, aimed at a variety of social and health problems (Sloboda & Petras, 2014).

Now, evaluation is a crucial component in prevention science and therefore in the development of preventive programs. In plain words, a prevention program that has not been evaluated is like a medicine without studies on its effectiveness. A prevention program without evaluation is potentially harmful, since, if it does not have positive effects, it can cause harm and the useless expenditure of resources can also be considered a harmful effect.

Due to the importance of prevention programs, they must be evaluated with a level of rigor comparable to other health interventions. In fact, preventive programs are considered health technologies, that is, procedures that must be safe and effective. The International Network of Health Technology Assessment Agencies defines health technologies as "An intervention developed to prevent, diagnose or treat medical conditions; promote health; provide rehabilitation; or organize the provision of medical care. The intervention may be a test, device, medication, vaccine, procedure, program, or system" (HTA, 2023).

Based on the above, there is a connection between evaluation and the guarantee of the rights to health and well-being since evaluation allows us to recognize which programs offer benefits, and which programs offer more benefits compared to others through the methodical collection of data. This is especially true when it comes to minors and the commitment of States to their well-being and safe development (UNODC, 2015). However, all people should have access to health and wellness promotion, as well as the best prevention programs for preventable diseases and disorders.

The Program Evaluation Process

Evidence is the set of tests and data that have been obtained through research and that allow us to support a theory or hypothesis. In other words, it is information that has been collected and analyzed to reach a conclusion based on facts and not opinions or beliefs. Evidence is essential for decision-making in many fields, such as medicine, education, and politics.

The evidence about a prevention program is not built overnight; on the contrary, the evaluation of a prevention program is a process over time if the following stages are taken into account:

1. Definition of a conceptual model. A prevention program is based on an understanding of why the event, behavior, or outcome you want to prevent happens. This representation is rooted in theories about behavior and the factors that influence it (Scoppetta, 2006).
2. Program design. Once a conceptual or theoretical model has been established, it is established how the factors that affect the behavior of interest will be influenced. Continuing with the previous example, it could be established that in a 2-hour session with role plays about social influence, the effect of preventing drug use would be achieved. The program can be understood as the set of activities, ordered in time, with an action protocol, with defined participants, with instruments and procedures for assessing their results.
3. Efficacy evaluation. Even if a program is based on a rational foundation, whether theoretical reasoning or evidence from other fields, there is no complete guarantee that the proposal will work. Before investing large amounts of money in massive applications and putting a large number of people at risk for counterproductive programs, it is advisable to test the program on a small sample but sufficient to draw conclusions and under controlled operating conditions. This is much better when you have at least one group against which to compare the results. This is called effectiveness evaluation (Brown et al., 2014).
4. Effectiveness Evaluation. Knowing that the program, under controlled conditions, achieves its objectives and does not have counterproductive effects, it is reasonable to apply it on a larger scale, evaluating its results in natural conditions. This is called effectiveness evaluation. It is also advisable here to obtain data from both the group that had the intervention and a group without the intervention (Brown et al., 2014).

Although it seems that with the four stages described, a prevention program already has sufficient evidence from the evaluation, the reality is that the evaluation of a program is a continuous process for the following reasons:

1. Social phenomena and their determining factors change over time. For example, in the case of drugs, new substances appear, legislation modifies the social status of drugs (such is the case of marijuana, legalized in different countries).
2. Programs must adapt in form and content over time. Today, for example, different forms of family and gender identities are recognized. This also applies to the case of programs that use audiovisual materials: It is not appropriate to maintain within a program materials developed decades ago, among other reasons because the people exposed do not identify with the uses of that time.
3. The way variables are measured changes over time, since they are also susceptible to social and cultural transformations. Therefore, it is necessary to re-evaluate the program over time to know if its results are maintained under changing social conditions.
4. When programs are applied in contexts other than the one in which they were initially developed, their adaptation and evaluation in the new contexts is required. In these cases, the implementation of the program as it was designed in the original context may be problematic and an "interpretation" of the program is required without losing its distinctive characteristics. This, today, is considered as important as proof of a program's effectiveness. It also happens that programs can arise in research environments, but when applied in real conditions their sustainability needs to be considered in economic and social terms. This is called "translation" or interpretation of knowledge and an entire discipline has developed around this (Brown et al., 2014; Lopez-Patton et al., 2015).

Types of Evaluation According to Their Purpose

The evaluation of a program can pursue several purposes. It is one thing to know if the program is being appropriately applied and another to know if the program is achieving the expected results. Of course, the first is a condition for the second. It is important to note that these types of evaluation are not mutually exclusive, and that they are often used in combination to provide a complete program evaluation. Furthermore, choosing the appropriate methodology will depend on the specific objectives of the program, available resources, and other contextual factors.

According to the above, different types of evaluations of the programs could be proposed once they have been designed.

Process evaluation: This evaluation focuses on measuring the implementation of the program and ensuring that it is being carried out as planned. Process evaluation includes measuring the quality of implementation, monitoring dosage (i.e., the number of times the program is delivered), identifying barriers to implementation, and analyzing fidelity (i.e., the ability of the program to maintain the integrity of the original model).

Evaluation of results: aimed at establishing the effects of the program on the participants or the target population. Outcome evaluation may include measuring changes in participants' knowledge, attitudes, skills, and behavior, as well as evaluating long-term outcomes, such as reduction in mortality rate or improvement in quality of life.

Impact evaluation: It has regularly been understood that this type of evaluation seeks to measure the effects of the program on the community or the population in general. Impact evaluation may include measuring changes in mortality rates, disease incidence, quality of life, and other indicators of social well-being. However, in academic circles and in the professional practice of contemporary evaluators, impact evaluation is one that seeks to establish evidence of the causal relationship between the program and the results of interest. For this, methodological designs and statistical methods have been developed with that this purpose is achieved. The impact evaluation would be within the highest level of evidence since it includes experimental methods as will be seen later (Gertler et al., 2017; Scoppetta, 2006). I will return to the impact evaluation later in this chapter.

Cost-effectiveness evaluation: This methodology focuses on determining whether the program is cost-effective and whether the benefits of the program exceed the costs. Cost-effectiveness evaluation may include comparing program costs with benefits, such as reduced disease burden and improved quality of life.

Levels of Evaluation and Levels of Evidence

A program may have been evaluated on a single or several occasions. On each occasion different evaluation methodologies may have been applied and different results may have been obtained in relation to their prevention capacity. In these cases, it is possible to ask how to assess the available evidence to know if a program works or does not work. Levels of evidence are a way of classifying the quality and quantity of evidence available about the outcomes of a particular program. Although there are different guidelines for assessing the evidence, we could summarize the levels of evidence for prevention programs as follows[1]:

High-quality evidence: High-quality evidence comes from rigorous research with an appropriate experimental design and a representative sample of the target population. These investigations may include randomized controlled trials (RCTs) and controlled quasi-experimental studies. High-quality evidence

[1] It is important to note that this classification of evidence is not the same as that used in the therapeutic or prognostic context of diseases.

indicates that the program has demonstrated effectiveness in preventing the targeted outcome.

Good quality evidence: Good quality evidence comes from studies that use an appropriate design, but may have some limitations, such as a non-representative sample or lack of randomization. Good quality studies may include pre-post studies and cohort studies. Good quality evidence suggests that the program is effective in achieving its objectives.

Limited evidence: Limited evidence comes from studies that have some important limitations, such as a small sample size, lack of randomization, or lack of control for confounding variables. These studies may include descriptive and observational studies. Limited evidence suggests that the program may be effective in preventing the targeted outcome, but more research is required to confirm effectiveness.

Conflicting evidence: Conflicting evidence comes from studies that have inconsistent or contradictory results regarding the effectiveness of the program in preventing the target outcome. These studies may include studies with inadequate designs or non-representative samples. Conflicting evidence suggests that more research is needed to determine whether the program is effective in preventing the targeted outcome.

No evidence: Lack of evidence means that there are no studies available on the effectiveness of the program in preventing the target outcome. This may be due to a lack of research in the area or the fact that the program is new and has not yet been evaluated.

It is important to remember that levels of evidence are not an absolute measure of a program's effectiveness, but rather are a guide to determining the quality and quantity of evidence available. The quality of the evidence expressed here may be affected by factors such as researchers' conflicts of interest or lack of rigor in practice. Therefore, randomized controlled trials must be carefully evaluated to establish their true value (Burns et al., 2011). Evaluation of prevention programs should include careful evaluation of the quality and quantity of evidence, as well as other factors, such as program implementation and appropriateness of the intervention for the target population.

When a program has different evaluations, it is possible to jointly analyze the data through systematic review and meta-analysis procedures. Well-conducted reviews and meta-analyses are considered a high point of evidence. Thus, in the guidelines for the assessment of evidence, it is considered that there is a hierarchy in the level of evidence so that systematic reviews would be in first place, with greater force if they include meta-analysis. The lowest levels of evidence come from case reports and finally from expert opinions (Balshem et al., 2011; Burns et al., 2011).

The Risks of Tampering with Assessments

The evaluation of the effectiveness of prevention programs is not free of risks as other fields of scientific activity are not. In general, these risks depend on the ethics of program designers or evaluators, which is manifested in the rigor with which they apply, or not, scientific procedures to establish whether a program works or not. The evaluation methodology implicitly is an ethical commitment to produce analyses with the highest degree of objectivity possible, reducing avoidable biases. In summary, the issue is that there can be different forms of manipulation of procedures and data, concealment of biases in evaluations, selective publication of positive results, among other forms of fraud. This is better known in other fields of applied knowledge, which has led to discussing the validity of the evidence presented in support of the effectiveness of health interventions. For example, Shedler (2018) criticizes that empirical research does not support claims that "evidence-based" therapies are scientifically proven and superior to other forms of psychotherapy. Furthermore, the author argues that empirical research shows that "evidence-based" therapies are weak treatments and that their benefits are trivial, few patients recover, and even the trivial benefits do not last. The author also points out problematic research practices that paint a misleading picture of the real benefits of "evidence-based" therapies, such as sham control groups, selected patient samples, and suppression of negative findings. Other authors show how the evidence in favor of certain interventions can be falsified in a crude or sophisticated way, usually after economic benefits (Goldacre, 2011; Silva Ayçaguer, 2014).

There is no 100% effective antidote against lack of ethics, which is in turn the result of deficiencies in training, among other factors. In the case of the evaluation of a prevention program and the assessment of the evidence, methodological training, the ethics of each interested party, controls and the institutional environment that encourages honest practices or not come into play.

Evaluation Trends

The interdisciplinary field of evaluation has grown in multiple expressions to the point where it is difficult to achieve a complete outline of the different branches into which it has diversified. A visit to sites such as betterevaluation.org that bring together a large number of accessible resources, and specialized publications such as the *Canadian Journal of Program Evaluation* or the *American Journal of Evaluation*, allows you to get an idea of the complexity of the issue today, so a summary of trends in evaluation runs the risk of being incomplete. However, it could be said that, in the twenty-first century, the evaluation of prevention programs has evolved towards greater use of evidence-based approaches and greater attention to the evaluation of long-term outcomes. From reading various sources and in particular "Evaluation in Today's World" (Thomas & Campbell, 2021) The following trends can be seen:

1. Evidence-based approaches: Prevention programs are increasingly being evaluated using evidence-based approaches, meaning that interventions that have been previously tested and evaluated are used. These approaches are helping to ensure that prevention programs are effective and that resources are used efficiently.
2. Evaluation of long-term results: Prevention programs are increasingly being evaluated for long-term results. This means that interest is increasingly trending towards seeing how prevention programs affect people's health and well-being in the long term, rather than just the short term.
3. Collaborative evaluation approaches: The evaluation of prevention programs is increasingly adopting collaborative approaches that involve all interested parties, including, in the case of interest here, professionals from the sectors involved (such as health and justice), researchers, patients or service users, and the community in general. This helps ensure that programs are culturally relevant and tailored to the needs of the community.
4. Use of technology: Prevention program evaluators are increasingly using technology to collect data and evaluate programs. Digital tools, such as mobile apps and online platforms, are being used to collect data more efficiently and to engage people in evaluating prevention programs.
5. Mixed Evaluation Approaches: Mixed methods is a research approach that combines quantitative and qualitative methods in a single study to understand and address complex research questions. In the context of program evaluation, mixed methods involve combining quantitative and qualitative data to better understand the effectiveness of the program and how it works in the real world (Creswell, 2014).
6. Adaptation approaches: The recognition of social, cultural, and economic diversity requires that the evaluation recognizes that programs must adapt to the contexts in which they are applied, even if they are based on solid conceptual models.
7. Equity approaches in evaluation: Increasing attention is being paid to social disparities and the need to ensure that programs are equitable and accessible to all. This means that evaluators are paying attention to how prevention programs may disproportionately affect certain groups of people and working to ensure that everyone has access to the same prevention resources and supports. Approaches such as developmental evaluation are considered very typical of these approaches.

Although these are evaluation trends that clearly go beyond seeking to establish whether a program achieves the expected results, these perspectives are partially contemplated by the agencies that finance evaluations or direct them. These entities usually adhere to schemes in which evidence is required from more traditional perspectives.

The following three examples could give an idea of how evaluation trends take shape in forms of organization and methodologies that are little known in Latin America.

Evaluation Systems

When we think about the evaluation of a program, we usually devise an evaluation experience, that is, a discrete event in time and activities that is executed as a concrete project from which the expected evidence is obtained. However, to develop what has been described in the previous lines, an organized effort is required, with the intervention of multiple actors, the application of different types of resources. So, the concept of evaluation systems can help think about the matter in a more fruitful way. An evaluation system can be understood as the set of evaluative activities carried out in the context of organizational structures that have a purpose in obtaining evidence that implies the permanence of the system at least in the medium term (Leeuw & Furubo, 2008).

Within an evaluation system, tasks can be organized and developed to collect evidence about prevention programs in cumulative, progressive, and adaptive evaluation experiences. One of the most important tasks of a prevention system is the increase in organizational evaluation capabilities. This involves managing increasingly complex evaluation processes while increasing the abilities of organizational members to understand and engage in evaluation processes.

The Realistic Evaluation

Although it was developed at the end of the twentieth century, this approach presents novel characteristics that contribute to a better explanation of why programs work or not. This explanation focuses on the decisions and actions of those involved. Rather than limiting the evaluation question to whether the program works, realist evaluation focuses on answering what works, under what conditions, and for whom.

The realist evaluation approach is a theory-driven form of evaluation, but is distinguished by its explicit philosophical underpinnings. Realist evaluators seek to identify the underlying generative mechanisms that explain how outcomes were caused and the influence of context. Realist philosophy views an intervention as working (or not) because actors make particular decisions in response to the intervention (or not). The "reasoning" of the actors in response to the resources or opportunities provided by the intervention is what causes the results.

Realistic evaluation begins with theory and ends with theory. In other words, the purpose of a realist evaluation is both to test and refine the theory of the program and to determine whether and how the program worked in a particular setting. Program theory describes how the intervention is expected to lead to its effects and under what conditions it should do so. The choice of data collection methods and analysis tools should be guided by the types of data needed to answer the evaluation questions or, more specifically, to test the initial program theory in all its dimensions. Realist evaluation is method-neutral (i.e., it does not mandate the use of particular methods). Typically, quantitative and qualitative data are collected in a realist evaluation, often with quantitative data focusing on context and outcomes and qualitative data on generative mechanisms. The term "generative mechanism" refers to the underlying social or psychological drivers that "cause" actors' reasoning (Marchal et al., 2012; Pawson & Tilley, 1997, 2001).

The Evolutionary Evaluation

The evolutionary evaluation[2] focuses on the social innovation process, continuous learning, adaptation, and improvement of the program or intervention. Unlike traditional evaluation, which focuses on measuring final results, this approach emphasizes the ongoing process of social innovation.

With this evaluation approach, adaptation to the particular needs and challenges of social change and innovation is sought. It is based on the idea that evaluative thinking, techniques, practice, and discipline can be beneficial for social innovation and that data collected systematically and properly linked to the objectives and strategies of users can make a difference, even in highly complex and open environments where objectives and strategies are evolving.

Evolutionary evaluation is based on systems theory and complex adaptive approaches, meaning it recognizes that programs and initiatives are complex systems that are constantly evolving and can be influenced by multiple internal and external factors. Rather than simply measuring end results, evolutionary evaluation works collaboratively with program stakeholders to continually monitor and adapt the program as it develops (MacGregor & Cooper, 2022; Patton, 2016).

Evaluation by Expectation of Results: A Proposal for Program Evaluation

The proposal that I describe below is presented as a complement to the evaluation processes and seeks to approach the solution of several problems that conventional approaches have focused on establishing whether a prevention program achieves positive results. Traditionally, judgment about programs is based on the positive difference between people who receive the program, those who do not receive it or receive another program. A program is said to work if the values of the outcome variable, drug use in adolescents, for example, are lower in the group that received the program compared to a group that did not receive it.

As seen in the previous pages, this approach is insufficient in light of today's evaluative developments. On the other hand, it is an approach that gives little

[2]The original name is "developmental evaluation". I translated it as evolutionary evaluation because it could be confused with developmental evaluation.

information to those who receive prevention programs developed in contexts other than those in which they will be applied. The difference in contexts occurs because prevention programs are developed in specific settings: a different country, a research group, or even a specific social and cultural context.

Typically, the adoption of prevention programs does not resolve questions about how many people (or families, or schools, or companies) have obtained positive results from participation in a program. An exact calculation of that number is not to be expected, but it is fair to consider that this would be important information. In the best of cases, it is accepted that the program "has evidence in its favor" because there were "significant differences when comparing the results with a control group." Although there are estimates for some programs of how much the return on investment is (in terms of how much money is saved per monetary unit spent), neither the program funder nor the beneficiaries are provided with information about what to expect from a prevention program in specific terms of how many people will have the expected benefit. On the other hand, this is not of interest in most evaluations, i.e., the evaluators look for differences between the intervened group and the observed group, without having an idea of the extent to which this difference makes sense. It is worth noting that the expression "statistical significance" is highly debatable and tends to be used in a ritualistic and thoughtless manner (Silva Ayçaguer, 2014).

On the other hand, "significant" differences between intervention and observation groups can be relatively small and significant, especially when the samples are large enough. This leads to paradoxical situations such as a truly effective program, when tested on small samples, may not show positive results. Thus, what is statistically significant may be non-significant in the sense that should matter most: the number of people benefited.

Consequently, when evaluating a prevention program, there should be an estimate of the proportion of people in whom the result the program promises would be achieved. What would be the source of this estimate? The answer is simple: from the data of the program itself. This implies that evaluators not only present the results of the differences between the groups, but also the proportion of people who had positive results attributable to the intervention. The publication of evaluation microdata, with due identity safeguards, contributes to this.

There are two application scenarios for the type of evaluation proposed here: First, those for the adoption of prevention programs developed in different contexts. This typically happens from high-income to low- and middle-income countries. Well, the recipients of the programs have the right or at least the reasonable expectation of receiving a program with the benefit that the beneficiaries in their places of origin obtain. If not, it is possible that the program will not be beneficial, not because of its formulation in itself, but because of problems in its adaptation. In these cases, it must be evaluated why the program failed, whether the failures can be corrected or the program definitely does not work in the specific context and should be abandoned.

The second scenario is that of the continuous evaluation of a program in the context of origin or in similar contexts. It is important to keep in mind that social, cultural, and economic contexts are not strictly homogeneous. For example, within any city it is possible to find many economic and quality of life disparities. For this reason, the inclusion of contextual information is very important in the evaluation of programs. In very restrictive terms, the location variable of the unit of analysis could be very informative if it contains a load of information that implies social, economic, and cultural characteristics. Then, in successive applications of a program, whether or not there are control groups, it could be evaluated whether the results are close to expectations.

Therefore, this evaluation approach could be called "by expectation of results," to the extent that the result obtained on each occasion is compared with a standard that comes from the data of the prevention program itself. The evaluation would lead to the explanation of the observed differences and valuable learning would be obtained from both the results below expectations and the results above expectations.

With the proposed approach, it is possible to establish that a program with evidence of obtaining good results may be below its performance in certain applications (Fig. 1).

Barring diminishing marginal utilities, it is to be expected that the more people who receive a good program, the greater the number of people who will benefit. So, cumulative evidence from a program could show how more people benefit as more of the population receives the program. But this benefit could also be below expectations, requiring explanation and eventual adjustments. Furthermore, with this approach the results of the programs could be predicted according to modeling that includes significant contextual variables.

This evaluation proposal integrates aa systematic vision since the evaluation of a program would require diverse evaluative experiences, it would also require enriched explanations of why results are obtained or not, but also of the extent to which these results are obtained.

Of course, this evaluation proposal has negative aspects, among others it could be noted that estimating the proportion of people who benefit from the program would be difficult in some cases, especially if the program is implemented in very diverse contexts. Additionally, this approach may require a greater investment of time and resources than conventional evaluation approaches.

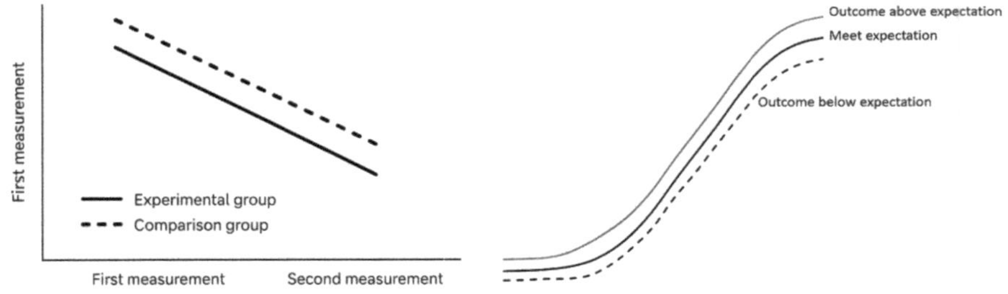

Fig. 1 Reasoning in conventional evaluation and reasoning in the evaluation of expectations of results. *Note*: The figure illustrates the differences between the conventional approach and the outcome expectations approach. The same program that programs with positive results according to a conventional approach turns out to be not so effective when its applications are compared with its own standard

Conclusions

Evaluation is a crucial component in prevention science and therefore in the development of prevention interventions. A prevention program without evaluation is potentially harmful, since, if it does not have positive effects, the useless expenditure of resources can be considered a harmful effect.

Evidence is essential in decision-making in many fields, such as medicine, education, and politics. In the case of prevention programs, the evaluation of efficacy and effectiveness is a continuous process that involves the adaptation and evaluation of the program over time, since social phenomena and their determining factors change over time. They must be adapted in form and content and the way of measuring the variables changes over time. Furthermore, when programs are applied in contexts other than the one in which they were initially developed, their adaptation and evaluation in the new contexts are required.

Program evaluation can have multiple purposes, such as measuring the implementation of the program and ensuring that it is being carried out as planned, establishing the effects of the program on the participants or the target population, measuring the effects of the program on the community or in the general population, determining if the program is cost-effective and if the benefits of the program exceed the costs. Choosing the appropriate methodology will depend on the specific objectives of the program, available resources, and other contextual factors.

Levels of evidence are a way of classifying the quality and quantity of evidence available about the outcomes of a particular program. Evaluation of prevention programs should include careful evaluation of the quality and quantity of evidence, as well as other factors, such as program implementation and appropriateness of the intervention for the target population. Well-conducted meta-analyses are considered a high point of evidence, and the guidelines for assessing evidence consider that there is a hierarchy in the level of evidence, with systematic reviews with meta-analyses being the strongest.

The evaluation of prevention programs is not free of risks and depends on the ethics of the program designers and evaluators, as well as the rigor with which they apply scientific procedures to establish the results. Additionally, lack of ethics can be the result of lack of training and other factors. In this sense, it is important to foster an institutional environment that promotes honest practices and adequate methodological training.

In the twenty-first century, the evaluation of prevention programs has evolved toward greater use of evidence-based approaches and greater attention to evaluating long-term outcomes. Collaborative approaches involving all stakeholders have also been adopted, technology is increasingly being used to collect data and evaluate programs, and quantitative and qualitative methods are being combined to better understand program effectiveness and how it works in the real world. Additionally, increasing attention is being paid to social disparities and the need to ensure that programs are equitable and accessible to all.

The proposal for evaluation based on expectation of results presented in this text seeks to complement the evaluation processes of prevention programs and overcome the problems that conventional approaches have focused on establishing whether a program works through the positive difference between the group that received the program and the group that did not receive it. It is argued that this approach gives little information to beneficiaries and does not consider the specific contexts where the programs are developed. Therefore, an evaluation is proposed that includes the proportion of people who would have positive results attributable to the intervention, which would contribute to a more precise and detailed evaluation of the program. This proposal would be useful in two scenarios: the adoption of prevention programs developed in different contexts and the continued evaluation of a program in the context of origin or in similar contexts.

References

Balshem, H., Helfand, M., Schünemann, HJ, Oxman, AD, Kunz, R., Brozek, J., Vist, GE, Falck-Ytter, Y., Meerpohl, J., & Norris, S. (2011). GRADE guidelines: 3. Rating the quality of evidence. Journal of Clinical Epidemiology, 64(4), 401–406. doi:https://doi.org/10.1016/j.jclinepi.2010.07.015

Brown, C., Mason, A., & Brown, E. (2014). Translating the intervention approach into an appropriate research design: The next-generation adaptive designs to effectiveness and implementation research. In Z. Sloboda & H. Petras (Eds.), Defining prevention science (pp. 363–387). Springer.

Burns, P.B., Rohrich, R.J., & Chung, K.C. (2011). The Levels of Evidence and Their Role in Evidence-Based Medicine: Plastic and Reconstructive Surgery, 128(1), 305–310. doi:https://doi.org/10.1097/PRS.0b013e318219c171

Creswell, J. W. (2014). Research design: Qualitative, quantitative, and mixed methods approaches (4th ed). SAGE Publications.

Doll, R., & Hill, A. B. (1954). The Mortality of Doctors in Relation to Their Smoking Habits. BMJ, 1(4877), 1451–1455. doi:https://doi.org/10.1136/bmj.1.4877.1451

Gertler, P.J., Martinez, S., Premand, P., Rawlings, L.B., & Vermeersch, C.M.J. (2017). Impact evaluation in practice, Second edition. The World Bank. doi:https://doi.org/10.1596/978-1-4648-0888-3

Goldacre, B. (2011). Bad Science: Quacks, Hacks, and Big Pharma Flacks. Emblem.

HTA. (2023). HtaGlossary.net | health technology. HtaGlossary.Net. http://htaglossary.net/health-technology

Leeuw, F.L., & Furubo, J.-E. (2008). Evaluation Systems: What Are They and Why Study Them? Evaluation, 14(2), 157–169. doi:https://doi.org/10.1177/1356389007087537

Lopez-Patton, MR, Weiss, SM, Tobin, JN, Jones, DL, Diaz-Gloster, M., & SMARTEST Women's Team. (2015). Translating evidence-based interventions from research to practice: Challenges and lessons learned. Translational Behavioral Medicine, 5(2), 233–241. doi:https://doi.org/10.1007/s13142-015-0307-2

MacGregor, S., & Cooper, A. (2022). Framework to Combine Mixed Methods Integration and Developmental Evaluation to Study Complex Systems. Canadian Journal of Program Evaluation, 36(3). doi:https://doi.org/10.3138/cjpe.71488

Marchal, B., Van Belle, S., Van Olmen, J., Hoerée, T., & Kegels, G. (2012). Is realistic evaluation keeping its promise? A review of published empirical studies in the field of health systems research. Evaluation, 18(2), 192–212. doi:https://doi.org/10.1177/1356389012442444

Patton, M. Q. (2016). Developmental Evaluation Exemplars. Guilford Publications.

Pawson, R., & Tilley, N. (1997). Realistic evaluation. Sage.
Pawson, R., & Tilley, N. (2001). Realistic Evaluation Bloodlines. American Journal of Evaluation, 22(3), 317–324. doi:https://doi.org/10.1177/109821400102200305
Scoppetta, O. (2006). Discussion on the impact evaluation of social programs and projects in public health. Universitas Psychologica, 5(3), 695–703.
Shedler, J. (2018). Where Is the Evidence for "Evidence-Based" Therapy? Psychiatric Clinics of North America, 41(2), 319–329. doi:https://doi.org/10.1016/j.psc.2018.02.001
Silva Ayçaguer, LC (2014). Biomedical research and its labyrinths: In defense of rationality for 21st century science. Díaz de Santos Editions.
Sloboda, Z., & Petras, H. (Eds.). (2014). Defining prevention science. Springer.
Thomas, V.G., & Campbell, P.B. (2021). Evaluation in today's world: Respecting diversity, improving quality, and promoting usability. SAGE.
UNODC. (2015). International Standards on Drug Use Prevention. United Nations Office on Drugs and Crime.

Orlando Scoppetta Orlando Scoppetta is currently the Director of Research and Evaluation at Corporación Nuevos Rumbos. He was trained as a psychologist, with postgraduate studies including a Ph.D. in psychology, a master's in population studies, and a specialization in statistical data analysis. Throughout his professional career, he has served as Director of Research at the Colombian Institute of Family Welfare and as Director of the Observatory on Drug Use of the Presidency of the Republic. He has also been an advisor and consultant to the Ministries of Health and Justice, as well as to UNODC, UNICEF, and IOM.

Overall Conclusions, Recommendations, and Projections

The prevention of the consumption of psychoactive substances has acquired sufficient recognition in the Western world to become part of the public policies of many countries. Thanks to systematic research, it has been possible to identify which strategies work best, in which contexts, with which populations, and in which age groups. Going through each of the chapters of this book allows us to see that developments in the field of prevention are associated, at least partially, with the level of economic development of a country or region, and its level of social organization. Thus, within the European Union, prevention is presented very differently between the richest countries and those with the lowest income. In Latin America, political instability is reflected in the absence of clear and far-reaching guidelines for working in this field; and likewise, a relationship appears between stability and progress in the desired direction, as is the case of Mexico.

This book shows a great diversity of approaches, but also certain common trends:

- What we call "the Western world" (the American continent, Europe, and Australia) tends to replace the punitive approach to drug and alcohol consumption with one of public health and human rights. Even though there are sometimes certain setbacks, most countries are issuing legal regulations that eliminate penalties for consuming substances, even when there are restrictions on doing so in public, by minors or pregnant women.
- In line with the above, there is an important movement in favor of the legalization of the so-called "recreational use" of certain substances such as marijuana. The first thing that was adopted was the legalization of the "medical use" of this substance, and many documents were published that apparently showed that there were a good number of health problems that could be treated with Cannabis derivatives (National Academy of Sciences USA , 2017), which gave birth to a multi-billion dollar industry. However, several systematic reviews (Martín-Sánchez et al., 2009; EMCDDA, 2018; Moore et al., 2024) have raised serious doubts in this regard. For this reason, we consider it prudent to reconsider these

A. Pérez-Gómez, J. Mejía-Trujillo (eds.), *Drug Abuse Prevention*, Advances in Mental Health and Addiction, https://doi.org/10.1007/978-3-031-99621-4

types of decisions and not proceed to promote behaviors that may have serious consequences at the level of public health, especially among minors.

- Another common feature is that Western countries tend to adopt an approach of analyzing protective and risk factors at the micro level (family, school, community), and controlling and managing social determinants (poverty reduction, environmental management, access to education, food security) at a macro level. While the former are factors that can be identified and managed by specialized institutions and organizations, both public and private, the latter must be addressed by state entities based on national policies.
- There is growing interest in evaluating preventive programs, but that is a long and difficult path that most developing countries have not traveled. It is easy to use discourses about "evidence-based prevention," but the reality is that the number of programs that meet the criteria related to having scientific evidence of the value of an intervention is, worldwide, few.
- Research addressing different aspects of the drug problem is relatively scarce, and most is carried out in the United States. The vast majority of works in other countries focus on the prevalence of consumption, either in national studies on the general population or the school population, or in micro-studies in small towns.
- Prevention programs continue to be very local and there is little dissemination, which prevents learning from culturally close experiences and making adaptations that, in the end, are more cost-effective than starting from scratch.
- It should not be forgotten that evaluation creates a problem: It "freezes" the programs, to which nothing could be changed without falling into what is called "lack of fidelity." As we showed a few years ago (Pérez-Gómez, Mejía-Trujillo and Mejía-Lynch, 2016), we live in a world that changes rapidly and it is not possible to use the same strategies when conditions have changed. A challenge will be to create preventive programs in which the principles, not the specific interventions, are evaluated: That would make them more resistant to the passage of time.
- Collaboration is essential in this field, and there are some signs that it is starting to happen. An example is "Evidencia Viva," a joint effort by the European Drug Observatory and some Latin American researchers to jointly analyze the experience of what is being done in the hemisphere. Another is the possibility of presenting research projects to entities such as the European Commission or the National Institute on Health of the United States, in which several countries could participate, despite the fact that in general the contacts between them, even when they are very close culturally, they are limited.
- In Latin America, it is essential to define state policies that insert preventive activities within a public health model, which has been happening for a long time in Europe. Likewise, it is necessary to give priority to investigative and evaluative processes.
- Although international policy is turning towards risk and damage reduction as a predominant element, it is important to reconsider this approach, since at the present time only in some countries, particularly in Europe, does it have a high relevance. In the others, where the basic steps have not been taken to ensure primary health care, it is necessary to first consider the offering of preventive, treatment, and social reintegration programs.

References

EMCDDA (2018). Medical use of cannabis and cannabinoids: questions and answers for policy making. Lisbon, Portugal. **DOI:** 10.2810/979004.
Martín-Sánchez, E., Furukawa, TA, Taylor, J., & Martin, JLR (2009). Systematic review and meta-analysis of cannabis treatment for chronic pain. Pain Medicine, 10(8), 1353-1368.
Moore, A., Straube, S., Fisher, E., & Eccleston, C. (2024). Cannabidiol (CBD) products for pain: ineffective, expensive, and with potential harms. The Journal of Pain, 25(4), 833-842.
National Academies of Sciences, (2017). The health effects of cannabis and cannabinoids: the current state of evidence and recommendations for research. Washington, D.C.
Pérez-Gómez, A., Mejía-Trujillo, J. & Mejía-Lynch, A. (2016). How useful are randomized controlled trials in a rapidly changing world? Global Mental Health 3. DOI: 10.1017/gmh.2015.29.

Index

A. Pérez-Gómez, J. Mejía-Trujillo (eds.), *Drug Abuse Prevention*, Advances in Mental Health and Addiction, https://doi.org/10.1007/978-3-031-99621-4

MIX
Papier aus verantwortungsvollen Quellen
Paper from responsible sources
FSC® C105338

If you have any concerns about our products,
you can contact us on
ProductSafety@springernature.com

In case Publisher is established outside the EU,
the EU authorized representative is:
Springer Nature Customer Service Center GmbH
Europaplatz 3, 69115 Heidelberg, Germany

Printed by Libri Plureos GmbH
in Hamburg, Germany